List of contributors

Dr Edward J Banham-Hall PhD MRCP
Consultant in Acute and General
Medicine
Addenbrooke's Hospital
Cambridge
UK

Dr Sian V Coggle MSc DTM&H FRCP
Consultant in Acute Medicine and
Infectious Diseases
Addenbrooke's Hospital
Cambridge
UK

Dr Sarah L Cowan BM BCh MRCP
Specialist Registrar in Acute Medicine
and Intensive Care
West Suffolk Hospital
Bury St Edmunds
UK

Dr James DH Goodman BSc MBChB
MRCP
Specialist Registrar in Clinical
Pharmacology and General Medicine
Addenbrooke's Hospital
Cambridge
UK

Acknowledgements

The third edition of Medical Masterclass has been produced by a team. The names of those who have written and edited are clearly indicated, and along with all these contributors I gratefully acknowledge the contributions of those who wrote and edited the first and second editions. This third edition is based on their foundations, and some of their material has been retained. But my acknowledgements must not stop there, because the Medical Masterclass would not have been published without the efforts of many other people. Naming names is risky, but I must name Claire Daley, who has worked as editor of the third edition with a wonderful combination of quietness and efficiency, and with an attention to detail that has made me feel triumphant if I have ever spotted a misplaced comma in a proof.

Dr John Firth DM FRCP
Medical Masterclass Editor-in-Chief

Published by:
Royal College of Physicians of London
11 St Andrews Place
Regent's Park
London NW1 4LE
United Kingdom

Typeset by Manila Typesetting Company, Makati City, Philippines

Printed by The Lavenham Press Limited, Suffolk

First edition published 2001
Reprinted 2004
Second edition published 2008
Updated and reprinted 2010
Third edition published 2018

ISBN: 978-1-86016-652-5 (this book)
eISBN: 978-1-86016-653-2 (this book)
ISBN: 978-1-86016-670-9 (set)
eISBN: 978-1-86016-671-6 (set)

Royal College of Physicians of London
11 St Andrews Place
Regent's Park
London NW1 4LE
United Kingdom
Tel: +44 (0)20 3075 1379
Email: medical.masterclass@rcplondon.ac.uk
Web: www.rcplondon.ac.uk/medicalmasterclass

Medical Masterclass third edition

Editor-in-Chief

Dr John D Firth DM FRCP
Consultant Physician and Nephrologist
Addenbrooke's Hospital
Cambridge
UK

Acute medicine

Editors

Dr Edward J Banham-Hall PhD MRCP
Consultant in Acute and General Medicine
Addenbrooke's Hospital
Cambridge
UK

Dr Sian V Coggle MSc DTM&H FRCP
Consultant in Acute Medicine and Infectious Diseases
Addenbrooke's Hospital
Cambridge
UK

Third edition

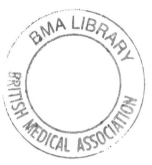

Disclaimer

Although every effort has been made to ensure that drug doses and other information are presented accurately in this publication, the ultimate responsibility rests with the prescribing physician. Neither the publishers nor the authors can be held responsible for any consequences arising from the use of information contained herein. Any product mentioned in this publication should be used in accordance with the prescribing information prepared by the manufacturers.

The information presented in this publication reflects the opinions of its contributors and should not be taken to represent the policy and views of the Royal College of Physicians of London, unless this is specifically stated.

Every effort has been made by the contributors to contact holders of copyright to obtain permission to reproduce copyrighted material. However, if any have been inadvertently overlooked, the publisher will be pleased to make the necessary arrangements at the first opportunity.

Contents

Preface

This third edition of Medical Masterclass is produced and published by the Royal College of Physicians of London. It comprises 12 books and an online question bank. Its aim is to interest and help doctors in their first few years of training, to enable them to improve their medical knowledge and skills, and to pass postgraduate medical examinations, most particularly the MRCP(UK): Part 1, Part 2 and PACES (the practical assessment of clinical examination skills that is the final part of the exam).

The 12 textbooks are divided as follows: two cover the scientific background to medicine; one is devoted to general clinical skills, including medicine for older people, palliative care and specific guidance on exam technique for PACES; one deals with acute medicine; and the other eight cover the range of medical specialties.

The medical specialties are dealt with in eight sections:

> Case histories – you are presented with letters of referral that are commonly received in each specialty and led through the ways in which the patients' histories should be explored, and what investigations and/or treatments should follow, as in Station 2 of PACES.

> Physical examination scenarios – these emphasise solid and reliable clinical method, logical analysis of physical signs and sensible clinical reasoning ('having found this, what would you want to do next?'), as in Stations 1 and 3 of PACES.

> Communication and ethical scenarios – you are presented with difficult issues that can arise in each specialty. What should you actually say in response to the 'frequently asked (but nonetheless tricky) questions', as required in Station 4 of PACES?

> Brief clinical consultations – how should you take a focused history and perform a focused examination of a patient who has a medical problem when there isn't much time? This section explains how to do this while working as a medical registrar on take, or in Station 5 of PACES.

> Acute presentations – what are your priorities if you are the doctor seeing a patient in the emergency department or the medical admissions unit? The material in this section is relevant to all parts of the MRCP(UK) exam.

> Diseases and treatments – concise structured notes that are of particular relevance to the Part 1 and Part 2 exams.

> Investigations and practical procedures – short and concise notes.

> Self-assessment questions – in the form used in the Part 1 and Part 2 exams.

The online question bank, which is continually updated, enables you to take mock Part 1 and Part 2 exams, or to be selective in the questions that you tackle (if you want to do 10 questions on cardiology, or any other specialty, then you can do so). You can see how your scores compare with those of others who have attempted the same questions, which helps you to know where to focus your learning.

I hope that you enjoy using the Medical Masterclass to learn more about medicine. I know that medicine is tough at the moment, with hospital services under unprecedented pressure and the medical registrar bearing more than their fair share of the burden. But careers are a long game, and being a physician is a wonderful occupation. It is sometimes intellectually and/or emotionally very challenging, but with these challenges come great rewards, and few things give more substantial satisfaction than being a doctor who provides good care for a patient. The Medical Masterclass should help you do to that, as well as to pass the MRCP(UK) exam along the way.

Dr John Firth DM FRCP
Medical Masterclass Editor-in-Chief

Key features

We have created a range of icon boxes that sit among the text of the various Medical Masterclass books. They are there to help you identify key information and to make learning easier and more enjoyable. Here is a brief explanation:

This icon is used to highlight points of particular importance.

Key point

A patient with a normal physical examination, a normal ECG and a normal echocardiogram is at very low risk of significant arrhythmia.

This icon is used to indicate common or important drug interactions, pitfalls of practical procedures, or when to take symptoms or signs particularly seriously.

Hazard

Acute lymphoblastic leukaemia may present in an identical manner to infectious mononucleosis.

Case examples / case histories are used to demonstrate why and how an understanding of the scientific background to medicine helps in the practice of clinical medicine.

Case history

A man with a renal transplant is immunosuppressed with ciclosporin, azathioprine and prednisolone. He develops recurrent gout and is started on allopurinol.

Acute medicine

Authors

Dr EJ Banham-Hall, Dr SV Coggle, Dr SL Cowan and Dr JDH Goodman

Editors

Dr EJ Banham-Hall and Dr SV Coggle

Editor-in-Chief

Dr JD Firth

The acute medicine section of the second edition of Medical Masterclass was written by Dr J Dulay, Dr SE Fairbain, Dr L Keating and Dr CA Eynon (editor). This third edition of Medical Masterclass contains entirely new material, but many sections from the second edition have been retained and updated, and we gratefully acknowledge the contribution of these authors.

Acute medicine: Section 1

1 PACES stations and acute scenarios

1.1 Communication skills and ethics

1.1.1 Cardiac arrest

Scenario

Role: you are a junior doctor on the cardiac arrest team.

Scenario: a 75-year-old man, Mr Tony Foster, has suffered a cardiac arrest on the ward. He was admitted 3 days previously with an inferior myocardial infarction (MI). Unfortunately, resuscitation attempts have been futile.

Your task: the nurses have asked you to speak to Mr Foster's wife and explain that her husband has died.

Key issues to explore

It is vital to find out what the wife knows already: she may have just arrived spontaneously without any warning of what has been going on; alternatively the nursing staff may have phoned to explain that her husband is very poorly and that she should come to the hospital immediately.

Key points to establish

> Get the setting right – ideally you need a quiet room adjacent to the ward where you are not going to be interrupted. Ensure that you have left your bleep (and mobile phone) with a colleague. Take one of the senior ward nurses as support (both for the family and yourself). The room should ideally have a supply of tissues and a telephone.

> Introductions – ensure you have introduced yourself and what you do; also introduce any nursing or other hospital staff who are with you.

> Ensure you have the correct family and know precisely who you are speaking to – many of us have had the misfortune to break news to a daughter thinking it was the patient's wife, or vice versa.

> Be explicit – explain what has happened: that the patient's heart stopped suddenly; that the cardiac arrest team was called; that attempts were made to resuscitate the patient; but that these were unsuccessful and that unfortunately Mr Foster has died.

> It is important to listen – give his wife time to understand and to ask questions.

Appropriate responses to likely questions

Wife: why has this happened?

Doctor: as a result of the heart attack, your husband's heart had become weaker – just after a heart attack the heart is irritable and the normal pattern of the heart beat can be disrupted, which can lead it to stop pumping blood properly to the brain and other organs.

Wife: what did you do?

Doctor: as soon as the team on the ward recognised that his heart had stopped, they called the cardiac arrest team. He was given oxygen and heart massage – pressing up and down on the chest to keep the blood moving in the body – and he was defibrillated – that's a special electric shock to try to get the heart beating steadily again. He was also given various drugs to try

to help, but I'm afraid that these didn't work. The damage to his heart was obviously too great.

Wife: would he have felt any pain?

Doctor: no – patients become unconscious very quickly as soon as this happens. During the resuscitation attempts he showed no signs of life and will not have felt any pain.

Wife: but on the television resuscitation is usually successful …

Doctor: yes, I know; but in real life the heart beat only returns in about 30% of people who have a cardiac arrest in hospital, and only around half of those survive to reach hospital discharge. I agree that things go well on the television more often, but unfortunately the figures are much lower in real life.

Further comments

Which deaths require reporting to the coroner (procurator fiscal in Scotland)?

> Cause of death is unknown.

> Deceased was not seen by the certifying doctor either after death or within the 14 days before death.

> Death was violent, unnatural or suspicious.

> Death may be due to an accident (whenever that occurred).

> Death may be due to self-neglect or neglect by others.

> Death may be due to an industrial disease or related to the person's employment.

> Death may be due to an abortion.

> Death occurred during an operation or before recovery from the effects of anaesthetic.

> Suicide.

> Death occurred during or shortly after detention in police or prison custody.

Who should be notified following a cardiac arrest?

> The coroner may be required to be notified (see above).

> The patient's general practitioner (GP).

> The consultant responsible for the management of the patient should be notified as soon as possible.

Who fills in the death certificate?

> Part 1 should be completed by one of the medical team caring for the patient. It should include the date of death and details as to the presumed cause. It has sections detailing whether information is available (or may become available later) from an autopsy, and whether the coroner has been informed.

> Part 2 is completed by a medical practitioner with at least 5 years of experience. Following the Shipman enquiry, the person completing part 2 will contact not only the person completing part 1 but also one of the nursing staff or another medical practitioner involved in the case to ensure there were no suspicious circumstances.

1.1.2 Stroke

Scenario

Role: you are a junior medical doctor on call for the wards.

Scenario: an 80-year-old man, Mr Anand Patel, has been admitted to hospital with a dense, left hemispheric stroke resulting in aphasia and a right hemiparesis. He has a background history of prostate cancer, left ventricular failure, atrial fibrillation (AF) and chronic obstructive pulmonary

disease (COPD). His Glasgow Coma Scale (GCS) score has fallen to 7 (E2, M4, V1), which is presumed to be due to an extension of his stroke. The consultant has reviewed the patient and feels that intensive care unit (ICU) care is inappropriate and that the patient should not be resuscitated in the event of cardiopulmonary arrest.

Your task: you are asked to explain to the family what has happened and why it would be inappropriate to attempt resuscitation in the event of cardiopulmonary arrest.

Key issues to explore

What preparations should you make before speaking to the family?

> Obtain as much information as possible about the patient's comorbidities and functional level before his stroke – in PACES scrutinise the scenario very carefully for details; in routine clinical practice look through the notes and speak to any staff present who may be able to give you useful information. This is essential, not only to inform appropriate decision making, but also in discussing the issue with the family. They are much more likely to accept advice from a doctor who clearly knows the patient – Mr Patel – rather than seems to regard him as 'just another old man who's had a big stroke'.

> The scenario states that ICU care is not appropriate, but if that is the case then what care is to be given? If the patient were to develop a chest infection are you going to try a course of antibiotics, or is only comfort care indicated? These issues may be spelled out in a PACES scenario; but in routine clinical practice it is very important to establish and agree among the medical and nursing team exactly what treatments will and will not be

given before embarking on discussions with a patient's relatives.

> What do the family know already, and what are their expectations? They may have expected Mr Patel to make a full recovery with supportive care.

Key points to establish

> Get the setting right – ideally you need a quiet room adjacent to the ward where you are not going to be interrupted. Ensure that you have left your bleep and/or mobile phone with a colleague. Take one of the senior ward nurses as support (both for the family and yourself). The room should ideally have a supply of tissues and a telephone.

> Introductions – ensure you have introduced yourself and what your role is; introduce any nursing or other hospital staff who are with you.

> Ensure you have the correct family and know precisely who you are speaking to.

> Explain what has happened – be explicit: the patient has had a severe stroke that has resulted in paralysis and loss of speech, and despite supportive measures his condition has deteriorated and he is now semiconscious.

> Explain your management plan – be explicit: you are going to ensure that he is comfortable, with enough analgesia (if required) and fluids to ensure that he will not be distressed. The priority is to maintain his comfort and dignity.

> Explain the limits of care that will be given – be explicit: that increasing the level of care is felt to be futile, and that ventilation or cardiopulmonary resuscitation (CPR) would not alter the outcome (families are often very relieved that their loved one will not be put through distressing 'treatments' for no effect).

> Listen – give the family time to understand and to ask questions.

Appropriate responses to likely questions

Relative: why has this happened?

Doctor: as a result of the stroke, he has very severe weakness of the right side of his body and he has lost his speech. After a stroke as big as this the brain sometimes becomes progressively more swollen, which makes things worse, and the patient becomes more deeply unconscious.

Relative: is he going to get better?

Doctor: I'm sorry to have to say this, but I don't think he is. He's had a very big stroke and things seem to be getting worse. It is possible that his condition may remain static, ie he remains unconscious and how he appears now for a prolonged period of time. However I think even this is unlikely and I'm afraid I think he's going to die.

Relative: is he in any pain?

Doctor: no, I don't think he is – I think he is too deeply unconscious to be aware of what's happening or to be in any pain. Our priority is to make sure that he is comfortable – and if we thought he was in pain or was distressed, we would give him painkillers to prevent him from being in any pain or discomfort.

Relative: if he gets worse, are you just going to let him die?

Doctor: the most important thing is that we make sure that he's not in any pain or distress. You are right that sometimes doing cardiac massage – CPR – and putting people onto breathing machines can be helpful. However, doing this is only kind and sensible if you have a condition that you can reverse with treatment and in this case I'm afraid that the effects of the stroke are not going to be reversible – ventilation and CPR would not have any effect on his underlying condition. We will ensure that he is comfortable and not in any pain – if you think he is at any point then please let us know.

1.1.3 Congestive cardiac failure

Scenario

Role: you are a junior doctor working as evening cover on a general medical ward.

Scenario: Mr Harold Wilson is 89 years old. He had a stroke 5 years ago and is a diabetic on insulin. He lives at home with his son, but has been housebound since his stroke. He was admitted 5 days ago with congestive cardiac failure. Medical therapy has been instituted, including oxygen, diuretics, fluids and vasodilators. There has been no response to treatment. He has become increasingly short of breath and is hypoxic despite oxygen. He has not passed urine for 4 hours. His GCS score is currently 8. He was reviewed by the consultant on the ward round who decided that he should be managed conservatively and not resuscitated in the event of cardiac arrest. His son was involved in the decision. It is now 9pm and Mr Wilson's daughter has arrived: she feels that her father should be on the ICU.

Your task: to explain to the daughter that transferring her father to the ICU would not be appropriate.

Key issues to explore

What does the daughter believe is likely to happen to her father? Why does she want him transferred to the ICU?

Key points to establish

> What does she know about her father's condition and his previous state of health? She does not live with him and may not be aware of these things.

> Explain what treatment has been given – he has been treated actively but has deteriorated despite this.

> Explain the prognosis – be explicit: her father is dying; and there is no treatment that will prevent this. Futile treatments (such as resuscitation or transfer to ICU) will not be given.

> Explain the management plan – her father will be given treatments to alleviate his symptoms and to ensure that he is comfortable and dignified (some people may be worried that a 'do not resuscitate' order means that no treatment will be given).

Appropriate responses to likely questions

Daughter: why isn't he on the intensive care unit?

Doctor: I'm sorry to have to tell you that your father is dying. He has been given treatment for his heart with oxygen, diuretics – those are drugs to get fluid out of the body – and other drugs to help the heart beat more strongly; but despite all of these the situation is deteriorating – your father's heart, lungs, kidneys and brain are all failing. There is no treatment that will reverse this – on the ICU or anywhere else; nothing that will alter the final outcome.

Daughter: is there nothing more you can do for him?

Doctor: we can try to make his breathing easier for him; we can make sure that he is comfortable and dignified; and we will ensure that he is not in any pain.

Daughter: you are only saying this because that's what my brother thinks.

Doctor: no, that's not true. We have spoken about things with your brother, and he does agree with our plan for treatment. But decisions about treatment are made by us and not by your brother or anyone else. We have made what we think is the right plan.

Daughter: *can I speak to someone more senior about this?*

Doctor: yes, I can arrange that. The consultant saw your father earlier today on the ward round. She is aware of your father's condition and the plan that I have outlined to you is the one that she made. However, she is not in the hospital at the moment. If you would like to speak to someone right away then I can find out if the on-call registrar is available to answer any questions you may have that I cannot answer, or if one of the doctors on the ICU could speak to you but I'm sure that they will tell you what I've already said. I'm very sorry. I'd like to be able to say something different, but your father is dying and we must make sure he's comfortable.

1.1.4 Lumbar back pain

Scenario

Role: you are a junior doctor on the medical assessment unit.

Scenario: you have taken a history and examined a 40-year-old man, Mr Chris Pitman, who called 999 with severe lumbar back pain. He is usually fit and well, but has a 2-day history of pain radiating down his left leg. There are no red flags in the history or on examination. Examination confirms a diagnosis of mechanical back pain. You have prescribed appropriate analgesia. On review, his pain has settled and you want to discharge him to the care of his GP. He is insistent that he needs X-rays prior to discharge.

Your task: to explain to the patient that no further investigation is needed at this stage and that he can be discharged back to his GP for follow-up with referral to physiotherapy if required.

Key points to explore

What is the patient's main worry? Why does he want further investigation?

Key points to establish

> The history and examination have given reassuring results: the pain is not sinister; there is no evidence of cancer within the spine (or any similar problem).

> Further tests are not indicated at this stage.

> There are simple strategies for coping with the pain.

> What to do if the pain fails to settle.

Appropriate responses to likely questions

Patient: *can you guarantee this pain won't come back?*

Doctor: no, I'm afraid that unfortunately I can't guarantee that. The prognosis for mechanical back pain is good, with 90% of sufferers recovering by 6 weeks, but recurrence is common.

Patient: *how do you know I don't have anything seriously wrong with me without an X-ray?*

Doctor: I'm afraid that an X-ray will not be helpful here. As I've said, there is no current evidence that this is a sinister problem such as cancer of the spine or anything like that. But even if it was, then it's extremely unlikely that a simple X-ray would show anything – you'd need other special scans.

Patient: *so shouldn't I have the special scans then?*

Doctor: no, I don't think so. The chances of them showing anything would be extremely small and they are not without risks, eg the effects of having radiation for the scans. However, if the pain continues beyond 6 weeks then the matter should be reconsidered. It is important that you arrange to see your GP when you get home, so that they can review your symptoms and see if anything further needs to be done at that time.

Patient: *is there nothing you can do for me?*

Doctor: yes, there is: I can give you some strong painkillers, some anti-inflammatories and some tablets to help muscle spasm. All of these can help and it is advisable for you to stay as active as possible – even simple exercises can help. Your family doctor could organise a referral to a physiotherapist if things don't settle down quickly.

1.1.5 Community-acquired pneumonia

Scenario

Role: you are a junior doctor on call in the acute medical assessment unit.

Scenario: Mr Kenneth Chang, aged 35, has been referred by his GP with chest pain, malaise, lethargy and a productive cough. His symptoms have been present for 4 days. He is otherwise fit and well, and takes no regular medication. He is a smoker of 20 cigarettes per day. Investigations have shown that he has right lower lobe pneumonia, and his CURB-65 score is 0/5 (the British Thoracic Society (BTS) guidelines scoring system, indicating a non-severe pneumonia in this case). You feel that his illness could be managed at home, but he thinks he should be admitted for treatment.

Your task: to explain the nature of his illness and treatment plan, including discharge with continued treatment at home.

Key issues to explore

What are the patient's concerns regarding discharge? Are there any problems with regards to discharge and recuperation at home? Is there a support network available if he is discharged?

Key points to establish

> Explain the diagnosis and that the treatment plan is in line with current national recommendations.

> Explore issues of smoking cessation in light of the patient's current illness.

> Give details of who he should contact if he has any concerns, and suggest reattendance if there are any problems.

> Explain follow-up plans after discharge.

Appropriate responses to likely questions

Patient: would I not be better off staying in hospital?

Doctor: no, I don't think so. The investigations have shown us that you have an uncomplicated pneumonia, and we have started the appropriate antibiotics and expect that your symptoms will improve over the next few days. I'm pleased to say that you do not have any signs of severe pneumonia, and your treatment can be safely carried out at home.

Patient: you only want to send me home because there aren't any beds in the hospital.

Doctor: I can understand why you might say this, but it's not true. If we felt that you needed to be admitted for treatment, then we would do so.

Patient: are you going to blame my smoking?

Doctor: yes, I am – at least in part. People who don't smoke can get pneumonia, but smoking damages some of the mechanisms that clear infection from the lungs, so as a smoker you are more prone to respiratory illnesses. Smoking will also delay your recovery from such an illness, so it is important to consider stopping seriously. If you want to try to do this, I would suggest that you discuss matters with your GP or contact one of the relevant support groups.

Patient: what if my symptoms deteriorate and I don't get better?

Doctor: as I said, I don't expect your symptoms to deteriorate. However, if things do not improve or if there are any problems then you should contact your GP for advice; and if things got really bad – which I am not expecting – then you could come back up to the emergency department, although I think it very unlikely that this will be necessary.

Patient: if I go home, will I need any follow-up?

Doctor: yes, if all goes well it would be sensible for you to organise an appointment with your GP to get checked over in a few weeks' time. They will listen to your chest and organise a chest X-ray to check that everything has resolved. I will write to your GP to let them know what investigations have been done and to ask them to arrange a repeat chest X-ray.

1.1.6 Acute pneumothorax

Scenario

Role: you are a junior doctor on call in the acute medical assessment unit.

Scenario: Mrs Diane Johnson, aged 36 years, is complaining of mild, right-sided chest pain. She is normally fit and well and is a lifelong non-smoker. On examination she is comfortable at rest and is not breathless. Her pulse is 85 beats per minute, her respiration rate is 14 breaths per minute and her oxygen saturation is 98% (on air) (normal range 94–98). On auscultation there are reduced breath sounds on the right. A chest radiograph reveals a small right-sided pneumothorax. You are happy to discharge her with no further intervention, but with a recommendation to avoid strenuous exercise (also flying and diving) until review, which you have arranged in 2 weeks. She wants further treatment and feels she needs to be admitted. Her husband is also very concerned.

Your task: to explain to Mrs Johnson and her husband that no further intervention is required and that it is safe to discharge her.

Key issues to explore

What are their concerns regarding treatment and planned discharge? Is an appropriate environment and support network accessible on discharge?

Key points to establish

> Explain the diagnosis, and the reasons for observation versus further intervention.

> Give advice on activity limitation, ie flying, diving and strenuous exercise.

> Explain that in the unlikely event of deteriorating symptoms, she needs to reattend.

> Explain follow-up arrangements.

Appropriate responses to likely questions

Patient: *why are you not going to treat me?*

Doctor: treatments are available which enable us to remove the air that has leaked into your chest, however these involve putting needles or tubes through the chest wall and so they are not without risk. We use them only when patients have a bigger pneumothorax than yours – so large that it makes them breathless – or the lung is very collapsed on the chest X-ray. I'm pleased to say that you have only got a small pneumothorax on the chest X-ray and it's not making you breathless. Therefore, the best advice is to wait: in 80% of cases it will get better on its own.

Patient: *what if I get more symptoms when I am at home?*

Doctor: it is unlikely that you will; but if you get more breathless or if the pain gets worse, then you should come back to the hospital immediately.

Patient: *if I go home, when will you see me again?*

Doctor: we will arrange for you to be seen in outpatients in 2 weeks' time, with a repeat chest X-ray. If there are any concerns prior to this, contact us or your GP. As I've already said, if you have more breathlessness or chest pain you should reattend immediately.

Patient: *what are the chances of this happening again?*

Doctor: you are right in thinking that if you have had one pneumothorax then you are at greater risk of having another one than someone who has never had the problem at all. It's difficult to put a figure on this, but the chances of you having another pneumothorax are probably about 30–40%. But the fact that you do not smoke and are fit and well reduces your risk of recurrence.

Patient: *we are planning to go on holiday to Spain in 4 months' time to celebrate our wedding anniversary: is this OK?*

Doctor: yes, it's important that you inform your travel insurance company – you should always do this if there's a significant change in your medical condition – but it should be all right for you to travel. The standard advice is that you should not fly for 6 weeks following complete resolution of a pneumothorax, and diving on holiday – which changes the air pressure in your lungs – is not recommended.

1.2 Brief clinical consultations

1.2.1 Palpitations

Scenario

Mr Kaveh Peters, a 54-year-old man, presented to the emergency department with palpitations overnight. His symptoms have now settled and he is keen to go home. Your task is to assess him and agree a management plan.

Introduction

Key point

Palpitations are a common reason for presentation to the emergency department. Patients may mean different things by the term 'palpitations' and so it is important to first establish exactly what sensation they are describing.

Palpitations as described by patients could refer to any of the following:

> an increased awareness of their normal heart beat

> a sensation of irregularity such as felt with ectopic beats

> sinus tachycardia

> a tachyarrhythmia – AF, atrial flutter, supraventricular tachycardia (SVT) or a ventricular arrhythmia.

Your aims in this consultation should be:

> to identify the rhythm if possible

> to look for any underlying physical condition or other precipitant that could have led to either sinus tachycardia or AF

> to identify any concerning features that could suggest a ventricular arrhythmia.

It is possible that the examiners will hand you an electrocardiogram (ECG) (which could show sinus rhythm or a tachyarrhythmia) either at the start of or during the consultation.

Beginning the encounter

Doctor: *hello, my name is Dr A, I understand that you have come in to the hospital because of palpitations last night: is that right?*

Patient: yes.

Doctor: *before we get onto the details of that, can you tell me if you have any major medical problems? Have you ever had palpitations before? Do you have any heart problems that you are aware of?*

Patient: [gives list (with doctor politely but firmly discouraging lengthy detail).]

Doctor: *and are you on any tablets or medications?*

Patient: [gives details (and will probably have been asked to produce a written list).]

These introductory questions will provide useful clinical context and may immediately give a clue to the likely diagnosis, eg known valvular disorder or cardiomyopathy, which may predispose to arrhythmias.

Focused history

Doctor: *tell me about the palpitations – can you describe exactly what you felt?*

Specific questions about symptoms that would be helpful in this case are:

> How did the palpitations start? A sudden onset and offset suggest a tachyarrhythmia (which could be AF or SVT).

> Have you ever had this before?

> How long did the palpitations last?

> Please tap out what the palpitations felt like. A clearly irregular rhythm would suggest AF.

> How did you feel at the time? Did you have any chest pain? Did you feel light-headed or dizzy? Did you pass out? Syncope associated with palpitations is a worrying feature that suggests a ventricular arrhythmia.

Questions to help you identify a trigger include:

> How have you been in the last few days? Have you been well or have you had any other problems, or any fever? AF is commonly

triggered by infection or by electrolyte disorders, which could occur with vomiting and diarrhoea.

> Have you had any chest pain / breathlessness? Pulmonary embolism (PE) may present with either AF or sinus tachycardia.

> How much caffeine do you have in a typical day?

> How much alcohol do you drink? Try to get a precise answer, 'not much' depends on the perspective of the patient.

> Had you had more caffeine or alcohol than usual in the previous 24 hours?

Focused examination

Some of your examination will be guided by the patient's answers to your questions (for example, if they have had a cough then you should also examine the chest), but the basic examination expected would be as follows:

Cardiovascular system:

> Feel the pulse – what is the heart rate now? Is it regular or irregular?

> Apex beat – is it displaced?

> Listen to the heart sounds – valvular disease (especially mitral valve disease) makes patients more likely to develop AF.

> Are there signs of cardiac failure?

> Ask the examiner for the blood pressure (BP).

Other relevant examination (if appropriate):

> Hold arms out straight – look for tremor suggesting hyperthyroidism.

> Look for a goitre, signs of thyroid eye disease, inappropriate dress for the temperature.

Questions from the patient

[Assuming that an ECG has shown sinus rhythm and that there are no

concerning features on history or examination:]

Patient: *what caused the palpitations?*

Doctor: I am not sure what caused them. The ECG we have done shows the heart to be in a normal rhythm now and I am reassured by the fact that you felt otherwise well when you had the palpitations. There are a few simple blood tests that I would like to do to check, but after that I hope we will be able to let you go home.

Patient: *what should I do if it happens again?*

Doctor: if you get the palpitations and feel otherwise well, like you did today, then you can wait a little while and see if they settle by themselves. If you get palpitations that are lasting longer, or if you have any chest pain, breathlessness or dizziness, then you should come back so that we can repeat the ECG and find out what is going on. If you are getting repeated palpitations, even if they are brief, then you should certainly let your GP know as that would probably require further investigation and treatment.

Questions from the examiner

Examiner: *what investigations would you do in this man?*

Doctor: I would definitely want to check his electrolytes including magnesium level (hypokalaemia in particular can predispose to arrhythmias), full blood count (anaemia can cause a sinus tachycardia or AF), inflammatory markers (infection can precipitate AF) and thyroid-stimulating hormone (TSH) (to exclude hyperthyroidism). If there was any concern about PE from the history (risk factors or symptoms) then I would want to exclude this either with a D-dimer or a computerised tomography pulmonary angiogram (CTPA).

Further investigations would depend on the history and examination findings but might include:

> 24-hour tape – if he is getting repeated episodes of palpitations then a 24-hour tape would be helpful either for diagnosis or reassurance, but if this was a single episode of a short-lived tachycardia then it is unlikely a 24-hour tape will capture an event.

> Echocardiogram – if there is anything abnormal on his cardiovascular examination or if the ECG has shown AF.

Examiner: *if he was now in sinus rhythm, but his initial ECG had shown atrial fibrillation, how would you proceed differently?*

Doctor: if the patient had had an episode of AF that had now terminated, then I would still want to check his electrolytes, full blood count and thyroid function. I would explain that alcohol and caffeine can precipitate episodes of AF and advise him to consider reducing his intake of these. I would also treat any underlying cause (eg a chest infection). I would request an outpatient 24-hour tape to see whether he is having paroxysmal AF, and an echocardiogram to look for an underlying abnormality of cardiac structure or function. If he were to have further episodes of AF then I would discuss anticoagulation and consider either a 'pill-in-the-pocket' treatment or a low-dose beta-blocker, depending on whether he had any structural heart disease and how frequently he was having episodes.

Examiner: *and if he were still in AF when you assessed him?*

Doctor: I would consider rate or rhythm control. If the time of onset was clear and within the last 48 hours, then electrical cardioversion would be my preferred option as long as there wasn't an underlying cause such as

infection. If the onset wasn't clear, or was more than 48 hours ago, then I would pursue a rate control strategy and also discuss anticoagulation. In either case I would request an outpatient echocardiogram and arrange follow-up with the results.

Further discussion

For details on rate control and anticoagulation in AF see Section 1.3.5.

1.2.2 Asthma

Scenario

Mrs Carrie Adams, a 21-year-old woman, presented to the emergency department with shortness of breath and wheeze. She was found to have a reduced peak expiratory flow rate (PEFR) and was admitted. A diagnosis of an asthma exacerbation was made by the admitting team, and she was treated with nebulisers and steroids. Her symptoms have settled overnight, her PEFR has improved to 90% predicted, and she is keen to go home. Your task is to assess her asthma and agree a plan for its ongoing management.

Introduction

Asthma is an extremely common and potentially lethal respiratory condition characterised by reversible airflow obstruction and bronchospasm. Although most patients with asthma have mild disease, some do not and require repeated hospitalisation, occasionally including intensive care support.

Asthma is a clinical diagnosis, supported by evidence of airflow obstruction that is variable over short periods of time. Over recent years, guidelines have moved away from using PEFR in diagnosis in favour of spirometry,

given the wider availability of this in primary care, although a normal spirogram when a patient is asymptomatic does not exclude the diagnosis. PEFR monitoring remains a useful tool in the management of asthmatic patients both at home and on the wards.

Clinical features that favour a diagnosis of asthma include:

> one or more of wheeze, breathlessness, chest tightness and cough – particularly if:

>> symptoms are worse at night and in the early morning

>> symptoms are triggered by exercise, allergens or the cold

>> symptoms are worsened by aspirin or a beta-blocker

> a history of atopy

> a family history or atopy or asthma

> wheeze on auscultation

> a low forced expiratory volume 1 (FEV_1) or PEFR

> an eosinophilia on full blood count (FBC).

Asthma as a diagnosis is less likely if patients report:

> dizziness, light-headedness, peripheral tingling

> chronic productive cough without wheeze or breathlessness

> repeated absence of wheeze while symptomatic

> voice disturbance

> symptoms only associated with colds

> a significant smoking history

> cardiac disease

> normal PEFR or spirometry when symptomatic.

Your aims in this consultation should be:

> to discuss the patient's asthma and key features leading up to this admission

> to confirm that the patient is well and safe to be discharged

> to formulate a plan to transition her care back to her GP.

It is possible that the examiners will hand you a PEFR chart either at the start of or during the consultation.

Beginning the encounter

Doctor: *hello, my name is Dr A, I understand that you came in last night because of a wheeze: is that right?*

Patient: yes.

Doctor: *before we get onto the details of that, can you tell me if you have any other major medical problems? Have you ever had an admission with asthma before? Have you ever been admitted to intensive care on account of asthma?*

Patient: [gives list (with doctor politely but firmly discouraging lengthy detail) – she has had occasional wheeziness before.]

Doctor: *and are you on any tablets or medications?*

Patient: [gives details (and will probably have been asked to produce a written list) – she has got a salbutamol inhaler, but uses it rarely.]

These introductory questions will provide useful clinical context and may immediately give a clue to the likely diagnosis, eg asthma presentation secondary to an identifiable precipitant.

Focused history

Doctor: *tell me about the wheeze and breathlessness – can you describe exactly what happened?*

Specific questions about symptoms that would be helpful in this case are:

> Have you ever had this before? (The patient may now remember previous episodes in more detail.)

> How long did the breathlessness last?

> How did you feel at the time? Did you have any chest pain? Did you feel light-headed or dizzy?

> Do you smoke?

> Do you have eczema or hay fever?

Questions to help you identify a trigger include:

> How have you been in the last few days? Have you been well or have you had any other problems, or any fever?

> Have you had any chest pain / breathlessness?

> Are you exposed to any dusts or fumes at work?

> Do you keep any pets at home?

Focused examination

General inspection:

> Does the patient look comfortable?

> Do they have a tremor? (salbutamol)

> Do they have nicotine staining or clubbing?

> Are inhalers, oxygen tubing or nebulisers visible at the bedside?

> Is there a pyrexia on the observation chart?

Respiratory system:

> Is the patient tachypnoeic?

> Check a PEFR.

> Do they have a wheeze?

Cardiovascular system:

> Feel the pulse – what is the heart rate now? Is it regular or irregular?

> Ask the examiner for the BP.

Questions from the patient

[Assuming that the patient seems to have suffered from an asthma attack without obvious precipitant, and from which she has now substantially recovered:]

Patient: *what caused the asthma attack?*

Doctor: asthma is a variable condition that comes and goes. Sometimes symptoms are triggered by allergies,

exercise or cold air, but sometimes – as in your case – we can't identify a specific trigger.

Patient: *can I go home?*

Doctor: yes, you can. Your symptoms have now improved and our charts checking your peak flow rate show that this has come back to normal. But I want to make sure that you are on the right treatment, and that you know how to use it. I'd like to check your inhaler technique, that you know what inhalers to use, and ensure you have a good self-management, because we want to avoid – if possible – you having to come back to the hospital as an emergency.

Patient: *I've got my blue (salbutamol) inhaler ... do I need anything else?*

Doctor: your blue inhaler is good for trying to relieve wheeze, but because you've just had an attack that's brought you into hospital, I think we need to start you on an inhaler that's designed to prevent attacks from happening. We want to try to stop this attack from flaring up again.

Patient: *will I need to come back to the chest clinic, or something like that?*

Doctor: I'm going to do a discharge letter for you to take to your GP. I'm going to ask them to keep a watch on things, and if there are more problems ask them to refer you to the chest outpatient clinic.

Questions from the examiner

Examiner: *suppose this woman had never been diagnosed with asthma before. What tests would you like to arrange to support the diagnosis?*

Doctor: I would like to arrange spirometry with reversibility testing, preferably while the patient is symptomatic. If reversible obstruction were present this would strongly favour a diagnosis of asthma. It would also be useful to arrange some routine blood tests as a finding of an eosinophilia would also be supportive, but further investigations are usually not necessary if the clinical picture is clear.

Examiner: *there is a standard structured plan for asthma management, do you know what this is?*

Doctor: step one is simply use of an inhaled short-acting bronchodilator such as salbutamol. Step two is addition of an inhaled corticosteroid. Step three is addition of a long-acting beta agonist. Step four is an Increased dose of inhaled corticosteroid or alternatively addition of aminophylline or a leukotriene antagonist. Finally, step five is addition of a daily oral corticosteroid tablet at the lowest dose required to control symptoms. These patients should be referred to a respiratory service for ongoing management.

Further discussion

For details on emergency management of asthma see Section 1.3.7.

1.2.3 Headache

Scenario

Mrs Methela Harrison, a 32-year-old woman, presented to the emergency department with a headache. She has also noticed some changes in her vision. What is the most likely cause for her symptoms?

Introduction

Headache is a common problem among patients presenting to the emergency department, accounting for around 1% of all emergency department visits. Most will have a non-sinister cause for their headache, but some will have a life-threatening diagnosis which it is important not to miss.

Features of primary headache disorders (ie headaches not associated with an underlying pathology) are shown in Table 1.

Secondary causes of headache that should be considered include:

> subarachnoid haemorrhage (SAH) – sudden onset, worst ever headache, may have associated neck stiffness and focal neurological signs, may present with loss of consciousness (see Section 1.3.29)

> meningitis – fever, photophobia, neck stiffness (see Section 1.3.25)

> giant cell arteritis – consider in over 50s presenting with headache; associated with temporal artery tenderness and jaw claudication

> venous sinus thrombosis – headache often associated with nausea and vomiting; risk factors include pregnancy, oral contraceptive use and dehydration; diagnosis by magnetic resonance imaging (MRI)

> raised intracranial pressure – headache that is worse on lying down, bending forward or coughing; associated with vomiting, papilloedema, cranial nerve palsies;

	Tension-type headache	Migraine	Cluster headache
Pain location	Bilateral	Unilateral	Unilateral
Type of pain	Pressure/tightening	Pulsating	Variable
Intensity	Mild–moderate	Moderate–severe	Severe–very severe
Effect on activities	Not aggravated by routine activities of daily living	Worsened by, or causes avoidance of, routine activities of daily living	Restlessness or agitation
Associated symptoms	None	Sensitivity to light or sound, nausea/vomiting, aura[1]	Unilateral autonomic activation (eg red or watery eye, nasal congestion, facial sweating, constricted pupil)
Duration	30 minutes – continuous	4–72 hours	15 minutes – 3 hours

Table 1 Features of primary headache disorders

1 Aura – occurs in roughly one-third of patients with migraine. Most commonly this is a visual disturbance and can be either positive (lights, spots or lines across vision) or negative (partial loss of vision). Other examples of aura include abnormal sensory symptoms and speech disturbance. These last for 5–60 minutes, are fully reversible, and can occur with or without the headache.

consider space-occupying lesions and idiopathic intracranial hypertension

> sinusitis – pain over frontal or maxillary sinuses with overlying tenderness

> medication-overuse headache.

Hazard

Red flag features on history or examination that require further investigation:

> worsening headache associated with fever or neck stiffness

> sudden onset headache reaching maximum intensity within 5 minutes

> new onset neurological deficit or cognitive dysfunction

> change in personality

> impaired level of consciousness

> recent head trauma

> headache triggered by cough, Valsalva manoeuvre, sneezing or exercise

> headache that changes with posture

> jaw claudication, scalp tenderness or visual change (suggestive of temporal arteritis)

> painful red eye, changes in vision (suggestive of acute narrow angle glaucoma)

> substantial change in character of patient's 'usual' headache

> new onset headache in a patient with an immunodeficiency

> new onset headache in a patient with a history of cancer.

Beginning the encounter

Doctor: *hello, my name is Dr A, I understand that the problem is that you have a headache: is that right?*

Patient: yes.

Doctor: *before we get onto the details of that, can you tell me if you have any major medical problems? Have you had problems with headaches in the past?*

Patient: [gives list (with doctor politely but firmly discouraging lengthy detail).]

Doctor: *and are you on any tablets or medications?*

Patient: [gives details (and will probably have been asked to produce a written list).]

These introductory questions will provide useful clinical context and may immediately give a clue to the likely diagnosis, eg a history of previous headaches that have followed the same pattern. A history of immunodeficiency or malignancy would immediately make you suspicious about a serious cause for the headache.

Focused history

Doctor: *tell me about your headache. What were you doing when it started?* [It is particularly useful to know about the onset of the headache – patients with a subarachnoid haemorrhage will be able to pinpoint the moment it started.]

Specific questions about symptoms that would be helpful in this case are:

> Have you noticed any changes in your vision? Can you describe what this looked like? When did this happen in relation to the headache?

> What is the pain like? Where is it and has it moved? How bad is it?

> Is this the first headache like this that you've had? If not, how frequent are they and how long do they last?

> Have you noticed any weakness or altered sensation?

> Have you had any other symptoms? Nausea or vomiting?

> Are there any activities or any positions that make the headache better or worse?

> Does the headache wake you up at night?

> What do you do during the headache? Do you use any painkillers for it?

> Has anyone in your family suffered from similar headaches?

> Ask specifically about oral contraceptive use (in patients for whom this might be relevant).

Focused examination

Your examination should be targeted at ruling out sinister causes of headache.

Basic observations (these may be available to you at the start of the station, but you should ask for them if not):

> BP

> temperature.

Neurological examination – check the following:

> neck stiffness

> brief neurological examination looking for any changes in vision, weakness or sensory loss

> fundoscopy looking for papilloedema, and noting presence/absence of photophobia (it may be that, because of the time allowed in Station 5, the examiners will indicate that you should not perform fundoscopy – but you certainly need to say that you would want to do so in this case).

Other relevant examination (if appropriate):

> palpate temporal arteries, particularly important if over 50 years old
> palpate over sinuses for tenderness (suggests sinusitis)
> look for rash.

Questions from the patient

[Assuming that the most likely diagnosis is migraine:]

Patient: what is causing my headache?

Doctor: from what you've told me, I think the most likely cause is migraine. This is a common problem and can be treated with painkillers. It is not dangerous, although it can certainly be distressing for people when they have the pain, especially if they have never had it before and don't know what is causing it. I will arrange for you to have some painkillers and hopefully you will then start to feel better.

Patient: don't you think I need a scan?

Doctor: [assuming that history and examination have not revealed any red-flag features requiring further investigation] from the story you have told me, and from my examination, I have not found anything that would mean that you need to have a scan. There is no test to confirm migraine. I realise that you are in a lot of pain, but I do not think that a scan will be helpful in diagnosing the cause of your headache.

Patient: is there anything I can do to stop getting another headache like this?

Doctor: some people find that there are particular triggers for their migraine, for example alcohol or particular foods, or tiredness, or associated with their periods. If you have repeated headaches like this, then it would be well worth you thinking about whether

there is anything specific that you had eaten or done before it started. If you find that you are getting a lot of headaches then you should see your GP as in that case they might start you on regular medications to try and prevent migraine.

Questions from the examiner

Examiner: how would you treat her if you saw her in the emergency department?

Doctor: I would give her simple analgesia – high-dose non-steroidal anti-inflammatory drug (NSAID) or aspirin is more effective than paracetamol – and consider a triptan for treatment of the acute headache. I would also give her an antiemetic if required.

Examiner: what features on history or examination would make you want to investigate this woman further?

Doctor: I'd want to investigate if there was anything to suggest a serious, life-threatening diagnosis … for instance, if the presentation could be that of a subarachnoid haemorrhage or meningitis.

Examiner: what would make you worry about a subarachnoid haemorrhage?

Doctor: the typical presentation would be with sudden onset of a worst ever headache. Patients will sometimes say that they thought they'd been hit on the head with a hammer. On examination they may have a stiff neck, and neurological signs ranging from coma to focal deficits.

Further discussion

Contraception in patients with migraine: the combined oral contraceptive pill should be avoided in women who suffer from migraine with aura. You should recommend that they see their GP to discuss alternative choice of contraception.

1.2.4 Postoperative breathlessness

Case history

Mr Justin Burton, a 71-year-old man with a past medical history of ischaemic heart disease and a 30-pack-year history of smoking, had an operation to remove a malignant colorectal tumour 2 days previously. He appeared to be making an uncomplicated recovery on the ward when he complained of breathlessness. You have been asked to assess him by the ward sister. What are the possible diagnoses and how would you manage him?

His most recent observations are as follows: temperature 37.4°C, pulse 84 beats per minute, BP 130/78 mmHg, respiratory rate 16 breaths per min, oxygen saturation 92% (on air) (normal range 94–98).

Introduction

From the outset, keep at the front of your mind the most likely diagnoses in this case: chest infection/pneumonia/exacerbation of COPD, pulmonary oedema, PE, or anaemia due to blood loss.

This patient's observations do not suggest that he is very unwell, but if he were to be so, you would conduct a focused history and examination while initiating treatment (see Section 1.3.2).

Beginning the encounter

Doctor: hello, my name is Dr A. I understand that you are feeling short of breath. Is that right?

Patient: yes.

Doctor: *before we get on to the details of that, can you please tell me whether you have any other major medical problems? I am told that you have had some heart trouble in the past, what was that? Have you had any chest or lung problems before? How far can you walk normally?*

Patient: [answers questions (with the doctor politely but firmly discouraging lengthy detail).]

Doctor: *and are you on any tablets or medications? Were any of these stopped prior to the operation?*

Patient: [gives details (and will probably have been asked to produce a written list), which are a shortcut for checking the patient's history of medical problems.]

These introductory questions will provide useful clinical context and may immediately give a clue to the underlying diagnosis.

Focused history

Doctor: *tell me a bit more about the shortness of breath you have now. When did it start? Have you ever had a problem like this before? Is it worse when you lie down? Do you have any other symptoms?*

Doctor: *do you have any chest pain … cough … feeling hot/feverish … palpitations? Any pain in your legs?*

Specific questions about symptoms that would be helpful in this case are:

> Do you have any chest pain or chest tightness? If so – when did this start? What does it feel like? Does it go anywhere else in the body? Is it worse when you breathe in? Pleuritic chest pain could be due to pneumonia or PE.

> Are you coughing anything up? If so, what colour? Have you coughed up any blood?

> Are you wheezy? This would support COPD but could also be caused by pulmonary oedema.

> Do you feel hot or feverish? Fever supports infection, but there are many causes and sources in a postoperative patient. MI and PE also typically cause a low-grade fever.

> Have you ever been diagnosed with a clot in your lungs or legs? If yes, ask for further details. When did this occur and why? Are you still on anticoagulation? Which one? Was this stopped prior to the operation?

> Any nausea or vomiting? Do you have any stomach pain? Any bleeding from anywhere? Shortness of breath may be due to anaemia from intra- or postoperative bleeding (although the observations given do not suggest this is likely in this case).

Focused examination

Basic observations (these have been given in the case scenario, but if not then you should ask for them).

Respiratory – check the following:

> Percuss – dullness indicates lung consolidation or pleural effusion.

> Auscultate – crepitations/crackles, particularly if bibasal, suggest pulmonary oedema. A pleural rub would be consistent with PE/pneumonia. Bronchial breathing would also suggest consolidation.

> Is there any wheeze? This could be due to COPD or pulmonary oedema ('cardiac asthma') in this man.

Cardiovascular – check the following:

> Heart rate and rhythm – sinus tachycardia is likely to be present, but is there an arrhythmia (of which AF would be the most likely)?

> BP and peripheral perfusion – significant cardiac compromise would result in a low output state with hypotension and poor peripheral perfusion (capillary refill >5 seconds). Pulsus alternans – alternate between large and low-volume pulse – may also be a sign in severe left ventricular failure.

> Jugular venous pressure (JVP) – an elevated venous pressure could be due to heart failure or PE.

> Added heart sounds and murmurs – these may suggest a primary cardiac pathology, although by themselves do not secure the diagnosis. In pulmonary oedema a 'gallop rhythm' with the addition of a third heart sound may be heard. Features of PE can include a third heart sound over the right ventricle, a loud P2 and right ventricular heave.

Other relevant examinations:

> Is there any leg swelling to suggest a deep vein thrombosis (DVT)?

> Palpate the abdomen and look for any overt signs of bleeding.

Questions from the patient

[Assuming that the diagnosis is not obvious:]

Patient: *why am I breathless?*

Doctor: at the moment I am not 100% sure what the cause is. There are a few possibilities. It could be that you have got a chest infection after the operation … that's quite a common thing to happen. It might be that you have too much fluid in the lung, which can happen in patients who have heart problems, which you've had in the past. It's also possible to get blood clots in the lung after an operation, but it's early for that sort of problem.

Patient: *what are you going to do?*

Doctor: the first thing I'm going to do is to give you some oxygen to ensure your breathing is as comfortable as possible. Then I'm going to organise some tests to try and work out what's going on … starting with an ECG, a chest X-ray and some simple blood tests.

Patient: *how will you treat me if I have got a chest infection after the operation?*

Doctor: apart from the oxygen, I will arrange for a physiotherapist to come and see you … after an operation it's very common for there to be some collapse of the bottom of the lungs, and physiotherapy can help to get the lungs opened up and get you breathing more deeply … and I will start you on an antibiotic.

Questions from the examiner

Examiner: *in managing this patient, what else would you like to know?*

Doctor: I think the key thing would be to review his clinical notes thoroughly, including the pre-admission clerking, the anaesthetic charts – looking for persistent hypotension that might have precipitated myocardial infarction, or difficult intubation with possible aspiration, the operation details – including estimated blood loss – and all the records since he's been back on the ward … his medication chart, his fluid balance charts.

Examiner: *what tests and investigations would you like to perform?*

Doctor: the first thing I'd want to do is to get an ECG, looking for myocardial ischaemia, also for a right ventricular strain pattern, right bundle branch block or the classical pattern 'S1Q3T3' that might support the diagnosis of a PE. I'd want to organise a chest X-ray to look for evidence of consolidation or pulmonary oedema. I'd want some blood tests including FBC to rule out significant anaemia, electrolytes and renal function to exclude renal impairment, and a troponin if a cardiac cause is possible. And depending on how ill the patient was, I may want to do an arterial blood gas.

Examiner: *would you check a D-dimer?*

Doctor: no, I think that a D-dimer wouldn't be helpful. I would expect it to be elevated anyway postoperatively. If I was concerned that the patient had got a PE, I'd want to do a CT pulmonary angiogram.

Examiner: *what features may you expect to find on a chest X-ray in a patient with left ventricular failure?*

Doctor: left ventricular failure will classically produce bilateral alveolar/interstitial shadowing, 'bat wings' – peri-hilar shadowing, fluid within the horizontal fissure, bilateral pleural effusions and cardiomegaly [Fig 1].

Examiner: *if this patient had left ventricular failure, what would be the possible causes and how would you treat it?*

Doctor: there are numerous causes of left ventricular failure (LVF), but in this situation I would be concerned about either excess iatrogenic fluid administration, withholding of usual diuretics, or intra-/postoperative MI. For treatment I would prescribe a diuretic (eg intravenous (IV) furosemide 40–80 mg) or an intravenous nitrate infusion. A low dose of opioid (eg diamorphine 2.5 mg IV, with antiemetic) may also be required.

Further discussion

Specific treatment will depend on the diagnosis: for PE see Section 1.3.8; for pneumonia see Section 1.3.9; and for exacerbation of COPD see Section 1.3.10.

1.2.5 Pleuritic chest pain

Case history

Mr Jonathan Chisolm, a 45-year-old man, has presented with pleuritic chest pain that started suddenly this morning. What is the most likely diagnosis, and how would you manage him?

His observations are as follows: temperature 37.2°C, pulse 78 beats per minute, BP 114/72 mmHg, respiratory rate 16 breaths per minute, oxygen saturation 94% (on air) (normal range 94–98).

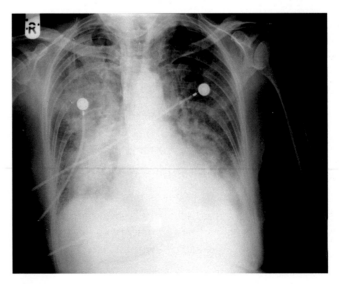

Fig 1 Chest radiograph showing features of severe left ventricular failure.

Introduction

Pleuritic chest pain is a common medical presentation with a wide differential that includes both sinister and non-sinister causes. The obvious diagnoses to consider are PE, pneumothorax and pneumonia/pleurisy, but keep in mind that this could also be musculoskeletal chest pain or even pericarditis.

Beginning the encounter

Doctor: *hello, my name is Dr A, I understand that you have been suffering from chest pain since this morning. Is that right?*

Patient: yes.

Doctor: *before we get on to the details of that, can you please tell me whether you have any major medical problems? … any heart or lung problems? … have you ever been diagnosed with a clot in the lungs or legs before?*

Patient: [gives a list (with the doctor politely but firmly discouraging lengthy detail).]

Doctor: *and are you on any tablets or medications?*

Patient: [gives details (and will probably have been asked to produce a written list), which are a shortcut for checking the patient's history of medical problems.]

These introductory questions will provide useful clinical context and may immediately give a clue to the underlying diagnosis, eg if the patient has had previous episodes of venous thromboembolism.

Hazard

Is this really pleuritic chest pain? Sudden onset pleuritic chest pain is most concerning for either PE or pneumothorax.

Focused history

Doctor: *tell me a bit more about your chest pain … when did it start? Where does it hurt and what does it feel like? Does breathing in make the pain better, worse or no change (or does it 'catch your breath')? What were you doing at the time? Have you ever had this before? Do you have any other symptoms such as shortness of breath, feeling dizzy or coughing up blood?*

Doctor: [if the patient has a history of venous thromboembolism then ask for further details] *you said you'd had a blood clot in your lungs (or legs) before – what happened then? What anticoagulant were you put on? Do you still take this?*

Specific questions that would be helpful in this case are:

> Are you short of breath? When did this start in relation to the chest pain?

> Do you feel hot or feverish, or had shivers and shakes? Has anyone in the family been unwell? Do you have a (productive) cough? Or a sore throat/runny nose? Any of these features would support a diagnosis of chest infection / pneumonia.

> Have you done any new sports/exercise/activity/weightlifting recently? Is there any chance you could have injured a muscle or rib in your chest? A history of unaccustomed exercise or injury would suggest musculoskeletal pain, also perhaps pneumothorax.

> Do you smoke (increases risk of PE, chest infection and pneumothorax)?

> Have you had any pain or swelling in your legs? Any such problems would clearly point to DVT with secondary PE.

> Risk factors for thromboembolic disease – cancer (or change in weight / bowel habit which could indicate an underlying malignancy), recent flights/immobility, family history, pregnancy / oral contraceptive pill (not relevant in this case). If they are an inpatient, then have they been on DVT prophylaxis?

Focused examination

This should begin with an assessment of the patient's general state: do they look well, ill, very ill or nearly dead (although in the PACES exam the latter possibilities are not likely)? Note the patient's vital signs: they have been provided in this scenario (ask the examiners for them if they haven't been) and show oxygen saturation 94% (normal range 94–98) which is lower than might be expected for an otherwise fit and well 45-year-old.

Respiratory – check the following:

> Palpate – reduced expansion could indicate pneumothorax. Localised (reproducible) tenderness is highly suggestive of musculoskeletal chest pain.

> Percuss – hyperresonance suggests pneumothorax while dullness suggests consolidated lung in this context.

> Auscultate – a pleural rub would be consistent with PE/pneumonia. Reduced breath sounds on one side would be suspicious for pneumothorax.

Cardiovascular – check the following:

> heart rate and rhythm

> BP and peripheral perfusion – hypotension and hypoperfusion (not likely in PACES) would suggest a massive PE/pneumothorax

> jugular venous pressure (JVP) – may be elevated in PE

> signs of right ventricular overload / strain – right ventricular heave, loud P2 and third heart sound are suggestive of PE

> a pericardial rub – would indicate pericarditis.

Other relevant examination:

> Is there any unilateral leg swelling to suggest a DVT?

> Lymph nodes, breast exam, rectal exam – an unprovoked PE would precipitate looking for possible malignant sources (but there would not be sufficient time for such examination in PACES, although it could be a cause for discussion with the examiners).

> Any obvious weight loss? Might suggest malignancy with secondary PE.

> Any features to suggest Marfan syndrome? Increased risk of pneumothorax.

Questions from the patient

[Assuming that the diagnosis is not obvious, but that PE is most likely:]

Patient: *what's causing this awful pain?*

Doctor: at the moment I'm not sure. There are a number of possibilities, but I think the most likely thing is that you have got a blood clot in your lung. I need to give you some treatment to try to stop any more clots forming, and organise some tests to find out if this is what's happened.

Patient: *if I have had a blood clot, then what have I done to cause this?*

Doctor: that's a good question, and I'm afraid that I don't have a very good answer. Some things do make a blood clot more likely to happen, such as a long flight, or being immobile for any reason, or having some medical problem, but none of these seem to

be relevant to you and for many patients we can't pin down a reason.

Patient: *I know that people who have blood clots have to have their blood thinned, is that right?*

Doctor: yes it is. If that isn't done, then there's a real risk that more clots can form, and this can be very serious, even fatal.

Patient: *but I know someone who had lots of trouble with bleeding after they were put on warfarin?*

Doctor: you're right that this can be a problem, but it's a matter of balancing benefits and risks. If we don't thin your blood, the chances of you dying from blood clots in the lungs are significantly higher than the chances of you bleeding to death if we thin your blood.

Patient: *I am not sure that I want to be on warfarin, are there any alternatives?*

Doctor: warfarin is still the standard option for treatment, but we do now have some newer drugs. These new drugs do have some advantages, the biggest being that you don't need to have regular blood tests for monitoring, but they've also got disadvantages, the main one being that you can't reverse them if there's a problem with bleeding. We will have antidotes for the new blood thinning drugs in the future, but they're not readily available at the moment.

Questions from the examiner

Examiner: *a CT pulmonary angiogram confirms a subsegmental pulmonary embolism (PE). What would you do?*

Doctor: I would first ensure the patient was clinically and haemodynamically stable, and that his oxygen saturations were within target limits. Then, unless there were some very strong contraindication – and I'm

not aware of any – I would begin anticoagulation with a treatment dose of low-molecular-weight heparin.

Examiner: *would you organise any further investigations for this man?*

Doctor: where a PE is clearly provoked, for example in a young patient following a long flight, then further investigation is not warranted unless there's some unusual feature. If there's no obvious cause for a first PE, then it's not such a straightforward matter. In any patient I'd have a low threshold for investigating, for instance, gastrointestinal symptoms, and I'd want to look at a chest X-ray, but most physicians would not recommend pursuing other investigations and imaging for cancer in the absence of any other clinical suspicion.

Examiner: *what advice would you give to the patient if you were letting him go home?*

Doctor: I would fully explain the diagnosis and management plan, and ensure he understood this. I would explain the recovery process and that he may find himself becoming more short of breath or tired quicker than usual, and therefore any exertion should be gradually increased and tailored to symptoms. Of course, he should be fully informed that if the breathing does not improve, gets worse, or he gets any chest pain, then he should immediately seek medical advice. Likewise, any leg swelling or bleeding would need medical advice. Finally, I would check that he was aware of follow-up arrangements with regard to his anticoagulation, and who to contact should he need advice.

Examiner: *do you give any standard advice to patients you start on warfarin?*

Doctor: yes, the most important things are to explain to them how it is monitored, and that the dose may need adjustment; that they need to get medical help if they have problems with bleeding; that they need to tell any doctor that they meet that they're taking warfarin; and that they shouldn't start any new medications without checking to make sure that they don't interact with the warfarin.

Further discussion

PE is a common presentation that all doctors should be comfortable with managing. Ensure you are familiar with all aspects from risk factors to diagnosis and treatment, including use of direct oral anticoagulants. Be aware of the differences in guidelines, diagnostic investigations, sensitivity of D-dimer testing, and treatment with low-molecular-weight heparin in patients who are pregnant.

1.2.6 Collapse of unknown cause

Scenario

Mr Timothy Collins, 70-year-old man, has been brought to the emergency department after being found on the kitchen floor by his daughter. It is uncertain how long he had been on the floor because he has poor recollection of events and his daughter did not see what happened. From the end of the bed you can see that he has a cut to the back of his head and one on his left forearm. What is the most likely cause of his collapse, and what is your management plan?

His observations are as follows: temperature 36.3°C, pulse 68 beats per minute, BP 112/64 mmHg, respiratory rate 12 breaths per minute, oxygen saturation 97% (on air) (normal range 94–98).

Introduction

'Collapse of unknown cause' is one of the commonest and yet one of the most difficult differential diagnoses in acute medicine. The case described here is typical: an older person has fallen to the floor, perhaps injuring themselves in the process, and sorting out what has happened and why is problematic because: (a) the patient is often unable to give a clear account; (b) there is a wide differential diagnosis of syncope (Table 2); and (c) the 'collapse' may not have a single cause – the blame may be attributable to the combination of a loose carpet, poor vision, an arthritic knee and recent introduction of antihypertensive therapy.

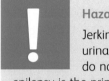

Hazard

Jerking limbs and urinary incontinence do not prove that epilepsy is the primary cause of a collapse.

Beginning the encounter

Doctor: *hello, my name is Dr A, I understand that the problem is that you've had a collapse: is that right?*

Patient: yes.

Doctor: *before we get onto the details of that, can you tell me if you have any major medical problems? Any previous collapses?*

Patient: [gives list (with doctor politely but firmly discouraging lengthy detail).]

Doctor: *and are you on any tablets or medications? And have any of these changed recently?*

Patient: [gives details (and will probably have been asked to produce a written list).]

These introductory questions will provide useful clinical context and may immediately give a clue to the likely diagnosis, eg new medication that has led to orthostatic hypotension.

Focused history

Doctor: *tell me more about the collapse … can you remember what were you doing before it happened? What did you fall onto and how long were you on the ground? I can see that you have a cut on your head and your arm, but have you any other injuries?*

Doctor: *have you had any other collapses, and were any of these witnessed?*

Table 2	Causes of syncope	
Type of cause	**Common example**	**Less common or rare example**
Neurologically mediated	Vasovagal syncope Postural (orthostatic) hypotension Situational syncope: > Urinating (micturition syncope) > Coughing (cough syncope) > Carotid sinus syncope	Situational syncope: > Defecating (defecation syncope) > Swallowing (deglutition syncope) > Postexercise/postprandial syncope Autonomic failure: > Parkinson's disease (some patients) > Diabetic neuropathy Cerebrovascular, eg subclavian steal syndrome
Cardiac	Cardiac arrhythmia Aortic stenosis	Pulmonary artery hypertension Atrial myxoma
Neurological	Epilepsy	Hypoglycaemia

Specific questions that would be helpful in this case are:

> Were there any preceding symptoms? Ask directly about chest pain, palpitations, shortness of breath, light-headedness (all would suggest a cardiac cause), nausea or sweating (typical vasovagal symptoms).

> Had you just changed position from lying or sitting to standing? Or had you been standing for a prolonged period of time? Both would raise the likelihood of postural hypotension.

> Do you recall events around the time of the collapse? Did you lose consciousness?

> Did you bite your tongue or were you incontinent? Were you confused afterwards, and – if so – how long did it last? Confusion or unusual behaviour after a collapse are typically features of the history given by witnesses rather than the patient, but they suggest epilepsy.

> Have you had any previous collapses that have been witnessed? If so, were there ever reports of changes in colour, pallor to flushing (suggesting a cardiac cause), or any funny movements or jerking limbs (suggesting epilepsy)?

> Any history of collapse with pain or unpleasant sights/experiences (epileptic aura)?

> Any new medication or changes in doses of existing ones (particularly of drugs that lower BP)?

In routine clinical practice you would wish to obtain as much information as you could from the patient's daughter, which is a point that you would make to the examiners at an appropriate juncture.

Focused examination

After briefly looking at the obvious injuries that have resulted from the patient's fall, particularly look for a short externally rotated leg from a fractured neck of femur, or for injury to the neck. Then proceed to:

Cardiovascular – check the following:

> Heart rate, rhythm and character.

> Postural BP – the scenario gives the patient's BP, but ask the examiner if a measurement of standing BP is available. In routine clinical practice, orthostatic BP measurements are recommended after 5 minutes of lying supine, followed by measurements each minute – or more often – while standing for 3 minutes. If the patient does not tolerate standing for this period, the lowest systolic BP during the upright posture should be recorded. A decrease in systolic BP ≥ 20 mmHg or a decrease in the level of systolic BP to <90 mmHg is defined as orthostatic hypotension, regardless of whether or not symptoms occur. You should be able to describe how this is done and ask for the results, but there clearly won't be time for you to do this in Station 5.

> Does the patient have a pacemaker?

> Heart murmur – in particular of aortic stenosis.

> Peripheral pulses – including auscultation of carotid arteries.

Neurological – check the following:

> Look for any focal signs, most likely attributable to stroke in this context, but also conceivably due to subdural haemorrhage in this patient who has banged his head.

Questions from the patient

[Assuming that the diagnosis is not clear cut, but that postural hypotension following a recent increase in antihypertensive medication is most likely:]

Patient: what caused me to collapse?

Doctor: at the moment, I'm not sure. The most likely thing is that your blood pressure fell a bit low as a result of the recent changes in your blood pressure tablets. I think we need to do a few simple tests to check out your heart, but I think it's most likely that the collapse was due to the blood pressure.

Patient: what tests do you want to do?

Doctor: I'd like to begin by doing a check of your blood pressure a few times, with you lying down and then standing up, to see if it falls; and I'd like to do an electrical tracing of your heart – called an ECG – to see that it's beating with a regular rhythm. I'd also like to do some blood tests to check the heart, also that there haven't been any problems caused by your collapse and lying on the floor.

Patient: I feel OK now; can I go home?

Doctor: I don't think that would be very sensible at the moment. Something reasonably serious obviously happened for you to collapse in the way that you did, and we need to try to find out what this was so that we can hopefully stop it happening again.

Patient: how can I stop it happening again?

Doctor: well, the first thing we need to do is to work out what caused you to collapse. If it turns out that it is due to the BP falling too low, we can cut back on your BP pills, and we can also give you simple advice about, for instance, taking a few moments when you go from lying to sitting, and then again before standing, and then wait a few more moments before starting to walk.

Questions from the examiner

Examiner: what further investigations would you perform in this case?

Doctor: further investigations would be aimed at identifying the cause of the collapse, and at ensuring Mr Brown had not sustained any injuries as a result of it. In terms of the cause, the key tests would be:

> ECG – to assess the rate and rhythm, also look for heart block or signs of ischaemia

> 24-hour ambulatory ECG – if there is a suspicion of cardiac syncope

> echocardiogram – to assess severity of any valvular disease, if clinically indicated

> CT head – may be required if there is the suggestion of a seizure from the history, or any focal neurology on examination.

In terms of injuries caused by the collapse and lying on the floor, the key tests would be:

> Urine – dipstick for blood and protein; if positive for blood, check microscopy for red cells. A positive dipstick with no red cells is caused by urinary myoglobin in rhabdomyolysis.

> Blood tests – electrolytes, renal/liver/bone profile, glucose, creatine kinase (CK), troponin I/T. A very high CK (>10,000 IU/l) with hypocalcaemia and hyperphosphataemia is typically seen with rhabdomyolysis. A grossly elevated troponin would indicate MI, but a lesser elevation would be non-specific.

> Imaging – depending on findings on clinical examination, X-rays may be warranted to, for example, check the hips.

Examiner: *how would you manage this case if the cause of collapse was confirmed to be orthostatic hypotension?*

Doctor: the most important thing would be careful review of any medication that might be responsible. This would obviously include antihypertensive medications, but other drugs, such as levodopa and dopamine agonists for Parkinson's disease, may be the culprit. Patient education with advice about simple measures, such as hydration and cautious changes in position, is important. Sometimes compression stockings can help and in extreme cases medication such as fludrocortisone or midodrine may be required.

Further discussion

Hazard

Seizures – a convincing history warrants treatment with antiepileptics, but these should not be given as a 'therapeutic trial' when the clinical picture is not compelling.

1.2.7 A painful joint

Scenario

Mrs Marianna Jones, a 45-year-old woman, has presented to the emergency department with a painful, swollen and hot knee. She has previously been diagnosed by her GP as having 'probable rheumatoid arthritis', but this has not been a problem for many years. What is the likely diagnosis, and what management would you advise?

Her observations are as follows: temperature 37.9°C, pulse 74 beats per minute, BP 150/78 mmHg, respiratory rate 12 breaths per minute, oxygen saturation 98% (on air) (normal range 94–98).

Introduction

Joint pain is a common symptom that may be a manifestation of a variety of rheumatic disorders, including those caused by inflammation, cartilage degeneration, crystal deposition, infection and trauma. It may be a localised manifestation of a systemic disorder. Consider the diagnoses given in Table 3 as you pursue the history and examination.

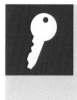

Key point

The first priority in dealing with an acute hot joint is to rule out septic arthritis.

Beginning the encounter

Doctor: *hello, my name is Dr A, I understand that the problem is that you have a painful knee: is that right?*

Patient: yes.

Doctor: *before we get onto the details of that, can you tell me if you have any major medical problems? Any previous painful joints? Any other joints affected now?*

Patient: [gives list (with doctor politely but firmly discouraging lengthy detail).]

Doctor: *and are you on any tablets or medications?*

Patient: [gives details (and will probably have been asked to produce a written list).]

These introductory questions will provide useful clinical context and may immediately give a clue to the likely diagnosis.

Focused history

Doctor: *tell me more about your knee … how long has it been painful and swollen? Have you had any trauma to the knee – fallen and banged it, or twisted it? Is it only your knee or are other joints involved? Have you ever had a swollen joint before?*

Table 3 Differential diagnosis of an acute hot joint

Frequency	Type of condition	Example
Common	Crystal arthritis	Gout Pseudogout
	Infectious	Non-gonococcal septic arthritis, caused by pyogenic bacteria – *Staphylococcus aureus* (70%), other Gram-positive cocci (20%) and Gram-negative bacilli (10%)
	Post-infectious	Reactive arthritis
Less common	Bleeding	Haemarthrosis
	Inflammatory	Other spondyloarthritides (not reactive arthritis)
	Infectious	Gonococcal arthritis (rare in the UK, more common in the USA and Australasia) Lyme disease TB
Rare	Inflammatory	Monoarticular presentation of RA Palindromic RA
	Other	Osteonecrosis (especially involving the hip)

RA, rheumatoid arthritis; TB, tuberculosis.

Doctor: *how is it affecting your daily life?*

Specific questions about symptoms that would be helpful in this case are:

> What is the nature of the pain? Is it there only on movement of the knee and improves with rest, or is it there on rest and movement, but eases after initial movement as joint 'warms up' (suggesting an inflammatory cause)? Is it there at any particular time of day or night?

> Is there stiffness in the knee?

> Any variation in the amount the knee is swollen?

> If more than one joint is involved, is it a symmetrical pattern?

> How are you feeling in yourself? Any fevers or shivers and shakes (rigors)?

> Any rashes or eye symptoms?

> Any ulcers in the mouth or 'down below' (on the genitals)?

> Medication – double check that the patient is not taking anticoagulants or systemic steroids.

> It may be appropriate to take a sexual history or ask about recreational drug use.

Focused examination

Given the concern to exclude septic arthritis, note whether the patient looks well or ill, and pay particular attention to the temperature (slightly raised in this scenario).

General – check the following:

> skin – for a rash

> eyes – for conjunctivitis or uveitis

> presence of tophi

> genitals – state that you would examine these for ulceration (which in routine clinical practice you would do in the presence of a chaperone, but which the examiners will obviously decline in PACES).

Knee – check the following:

> inspect and palpate for swelling, erythema, synovial effusion and warmth, comparing the affected joint with the contralateral one

> check motion – active and passive

> palpate for crepitus with passive movement.

Questions from the patient

[Assuming that the diagnosis is not clear cut, but that the knee is the only joint that is obviously involved:]

Patient: *what's causing the problem with my knee?*

Doctor: at the moment, I'm not sure. The first thing that we need to do is to make sure that it's not caused by an infection in the joint.

Patient: *how are you going to do that?*

Doctor: as you can see yourself, the joint is swollen. That's because it has fluid in it. The way to tell if there's an infection in it is for me to take a small sample of that fluid away with a fine needle – a bit like having a blood test done – and then get the fluid tested in the laboratory.

Patient: *my family doctor thought I might have rheumatoid arthritis; is that what you think?*

Doctor: it would be unusual for rheumatoid arthritis to present this way, with a single large joint that is swollen. It more commonly presents with lots (5 or more) of joints that are swollen. So I think it's unlikely, but I can't definitely rule it out at this stage, and we will investigate for this.

Patient: *if this could be an infection, do I need antibiotics now?*

Doctor: I can understand why you say that, but the first thing we need to do is to work out if this is an infection in the joint, and – if so – try and establish which particular bacteria are causing it. To do this we need to take some of the fluid from your knee and analyse it in the laboratory, and taking the fluid may also help with the pain as it will relieve some of the pressure on the joint.

Patient: *if it is an infection, will antibiotics sort it out?*

Doctor: they will certainly be a crucial part of the treatment, but if the tests show that you do have an infection we will ask the orthopaedic surgeons to see you. It may be that an operation will be needed to wash out the knee.

Questions from the examiner

Examiner: *what investigations are you going to perform?*

Doctor: the crucial investigation in this case is to obtain an aspirate of synovial fluid from the knee joint for microscopy and culture. The key things on microscopy would be to look at the white blood cell count, a Gram stain to look for bacteria, and polarising microscopy to look for crystals of gout or pseudogout and culture.

Examiner: *would any other tests be helpful?*

Doctor: blood cultures should be taken in all cases, a clotting screen performed if there is haemarthrosis, and the serum uric acid if there are crystals of gout in the joint. Other tests don't often provide useful information in patients with a single hot joint: the white blood cell count may be raised in infection; elevation of inflammatory markers (erythrocyte sedimentation rate and C-reactive protein) is non-specific; testing for

autoantibodies is rarely revealing; and joint radiographs are usually unhelpful, although chondrocalcinosis may be seen in pseudogout.

Examiner: *how will you manage this patient?*

Doctor: specific treatment will depend on the underlying cause, such as antibiotics and joint washout if this is a septic arthritis, and all patients will need adequate analgesia. Non-steroidal anti-inflammatory drugs should initially be given at their maximum recommended dosage until symptoms improve, after which they should be tapered gradually over several days. Appropriate joint support and positioning can also be very helpful. Some patients will also need strong analgesics.

Examiner: *supposing the diagnosis turned out to be an acute attack of gout, how would you treat that?*

Doctor: the options for dealing with an acute attack are non-steroidals, colchicine and prednisolone. Giving steroid into the joint can be very effective.

Further discussion

Findings on aspiration of synovial fluid are shown in Table 4.

1.2.8 Weight loss

Scenario

Mrs Tabitha Jones, a 47-year-old woman, has been referred by her GP to a general medical outpatient clinic on account of the fact that she has lost 5 kg in weight. What is the likely diagnosis, and how would you investigate?

Her observations are as follows: temperature 37.3°C, pulse 92 beats per minute, BP 110/64 mmHg, respiratory rate 14 breaths per minute, oxygen saturation 97% (on air) (normal range 94–98).

Introduction

The challenge in this scenario is that you are provided with a very non-specific symptom – weight loss – and no other strong clues as to the underlying cause. It is therefore very important to start with open questions about the patient's symptoms in the hope that the answers to these will provide direction. An obvious possibility (in routine clinical practice, and certainly in the context of PACES) is thyrotoxicosis, and it will also be important to screen for features that might suggest malignancy.

Table 4	Characteristics of synovial fluid in various conditions		
Condition	Macroscopic appearance	WCC (/mm^3)	Polymorphonuclear neutrophils
Normal	Clear	0–200	<10%
Non-inflammatory	Clear	200–2,000	<20%
Inflammatory	Slightly turbid	2,000–50,000	20–70%
Pyoarthrosis	Turbid	>50,000	>70%
WCC, white cell count.			

Beginning the encounter

Doctor: *hello, my name is Dr A, I understand that you have come to clinic today because of weight loss: is that right?*

Patient: yes.

Doctor: *could you tell me about that and any other symptoms you've noticed at the same time?*

Patient: [gives additional clues that may well make the working diagnosis clear (with doctor politely but firmly discouraging lengthy detail).]

Doctor: *and are you on any tablets or medications?*

Patient: [gives details (and will probably have been asked to produce a written list).]

These introductory questions will provide useful clinical context and may immediately give a clue to the likely diagnosis, eg new thyrotoxicosis or a recurrence of previously treated thyrotoxicosis.

Focused history

Doctor: please tell me more about the weight loss.

> Have you ever had this before?

> When did it start?

> How much weight have you lost? [The scenario says 5 kg, but it would be sensible to check.]

> Have you been dieting or trying to lose weight? [The overweight patient who has lost weight by dieting or exercise is to be congratulated and not investigated for weight loss!]

General screening – specific questions that would be helpful in this case include:

> Is your appetite OK? Anorexia would increase concern about malignancy.

> Have you had any problems with your breathing or your chest? Or with indigestion, abdominal pain, swelling of your abdomen, or your bowels? Or any problems with the water works? Any positive answers should be explored.

> Do you smoke? Increases the risk of malignancy.

Considering the diagnosis of thyrotoxicosis – check the following:

> nervousness and irritability; anxiety; insomnia

> perspiration/sweating

> palpitations – has your heart been racing at all?

> shakiness – do you find that you shake the cup when you try to have a drink?

> muscle weakness

> diarrhoea

> have you had any problems with diabetes or other gland problems in the past?

> has anybody in your family had thyroid disease?

Considering the diagnosis of lymphoma – check the following:

> fevers and/or drenching sweats

> itching.

Further symptoms should also be discussed if the patient you are assessing has obvious clinical evidence of thyroid eye disease or a visible goitre.

> Any trouble with pain or soreness of the eyes?

> Any problem with breathing? Do you make a sound like a wheeze when you're exercising? (Which might be due to stridor.)

Focused examination

This will clearly be guided by the history, but the basic approach – assuming that there are no pointers to primarily respiratory or gastrointestinal pathology – should be as follows:

General inspection:

> Does the patient look well, or ill?

> Do they have a tremor?

> Do they have any thyroid acropachy?

> Do they have any pretibial myxoedema?

Neck:

> Check for a goitre.

> Check for a thyroid bruit.

Eyes:

> Check for proptosis, exophthalmos and lid lag.

Cardiovascular system:

> Feel the pulse – what is the heart rate now? Is it regular or irregular?

Questions from the patient

[Assuming that the diagnosis is very likely to be thyrotoxicosis, with examination revealing a small smooth goitre:]

Patient: *why have I lost weight?*

Doctor: I think that the most likely reason for this is that you have got a condition called hyperthyroidism, which is where the thyroid gland in your neck becomes overactive and causes your metabolism to speed up. In the first instance we will check this with a simple blood test.

Patient: *what blood tests will you do?*

Doctor: the first thing will be to check that the thyroid gland really is overactive. We'll do this by measuring the level of thyroid hormones in the blood, and also the thing in the blood that tells the thyroid gland how hard to work. We will also do another blood test that might tell us why the thyroid has become overactive.

Patient: *if my thyroid is overactive what treatment will I need?*

Doctor: the treatment will begin with tablets that reduce the thyroid overactivity. It takes a few weeks for these to work, and so if symptoms like the heart racing or your hands shaking are a significant problem, we can also give you a tablet called a beta-blocker to help while we wait for the thyroid medication to take effect.

Questions from the examiner

Examiner: *what is the most likely cause of her hyperthyroidism, and how would you investigate for it?*

Doctor: I think she's most likely to have Graves' disease. Apart from checking her T4 and TSH, I'd want to check for thyroid autoantibodies, in particular looking for thyroid-stimulating immunoglobulin.

Examiner: *what would you do if this patient had a normal T4 level and a reduced TSH?*

Doctor: the next step would be to test their T3 level. The patient's history is very suggestive of thyrotoxicosis and it is possible that she has T3 thyrotoxicosis causing her symptoms.

Examiner: *what are first-line treatments for hyperthyroidism?*

Doctor: the first-line treatment is with either carbimazole or propylthiouracil to reduce thyroid overactivity.

This could be managed either with a block-and-replace regimen, or with a reducing dose regimen. Beta-blockers such as propranolol can be used to improve symptoms such as tremor and palpitations.

Examiner: *and if the patient relapses after treatment with carbimazole, what are the treatment options?*

Doctor: either thyroidectomy or radioactive iodine, with lifelong treatment with thyroxine afterwards.

Further discussion

Key point

Hyperthyroidism is an extremely common condition with a myriad of clinical presentations that can lead to a delay in diagnosis simply due to the heterogeneity of the symptoms that it may cause.

1.3 Acute scenarios

1.3.1 Cardiac arrest

Case history

A 75-year-old man is found collapsed in bed on the ward. He was admitted 3 days previously with an inferior myocardial infarction (MI). You are called as a member of the cardiac arrest team.

Introduction

Confirmation of cardiac arrest

Key point

Confirmation of cardiac arrest:

> Shake the patient and shout at them – 'Are you OK? Can you hear me?'

> If there is no response, then shout for help.

> Open the airway – use the head-tilt, chin-lift method (or if trauma is suspected, use the jaw thrust method).

> Check for signs of normal breathing and feel for the carotid pulse (<10 seconds).

> If the patient has no signs of life, is not breathing, has no pulse or if there is any doubt:

>> send someone for help; or if you are on your own, leave the victim and alert the resuscitation team (2222) / ambulance service (999)

>> start chest compressions, combining them with rescue breathing at a rate of 30:2.

Hazard

> Checking the carotid pulse is an inaccurate method of confirming cardiac arrest: if in doubt commence CPR.

> Agonal breaths are common immediately following sudden cardiac arrest and should not delay commencement of CPR.

Who should be resuscitated?

Cardiorespiratory arrest is common to all causes of death, but CPR should only be attempted if there is a potentially reversible cause for the arrest. An attempt should be made to resuscitate all patients unless a decision not to attempt resuscitation (do not resuscitate (DNR) order) has been written in the nursing and medical notes. In an acute situation, decisions about CPR should be made by the most senior medical person present at the time, and discussed with the consultant in charge of the case at the earliest opportunity. If the clinical condition of a patient alters, then decisions about CPR and/or DNR orders should be reconsidered. It is good practice to discuss CPR decisions with both the patient and their relatives if possible.

> **! Hazard**
>
> Many patients are concerned that a DNR order implies that nothing will be done – even to the extent of withholding analgesia and fluids in the event of their decline. They must be strongly reassured that this is not so.

Management

Basic life support

Basic life support (BLS) comprises initial assessment, maintenance of a patent airway, rescue breathing and closed-chest compressions (see Fig 2). The primary objective is to provide sufficient oxygenated blood to the brain and heart until definitive therapy can be applied and a spontaneous circulation re-established. BLS is a holding method only, but it at least doubles the chances of survival if

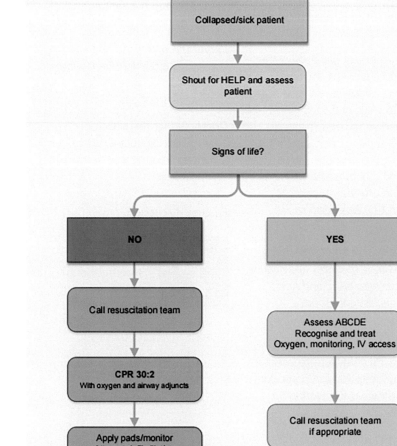

Resuscitation Council (UK) GUIDELINES 2015   **In-hospital Resuscitation**

Fig 2 Resuscitation Council UK 2015 guidelines for single rescuer in hospital BLS. (Reproduced with the kind permission of the Resuscitation Council (UK).) CPR, cardiopulmonary resuscitation.

applied between the time of collapse and first defibrillation.

Cardiac output during CPR ranges from a quarter to a third of normal. Diastolic BP and consequently coronary perfusion pressure falls rapidly after the first few minutes of CPR.

Advanced life support

Advanced life support (ALS) consists of definitive airway management and the use of drugs and defibrillation to attempt to re-establish a spontaneous cardiac output (Fig 3).

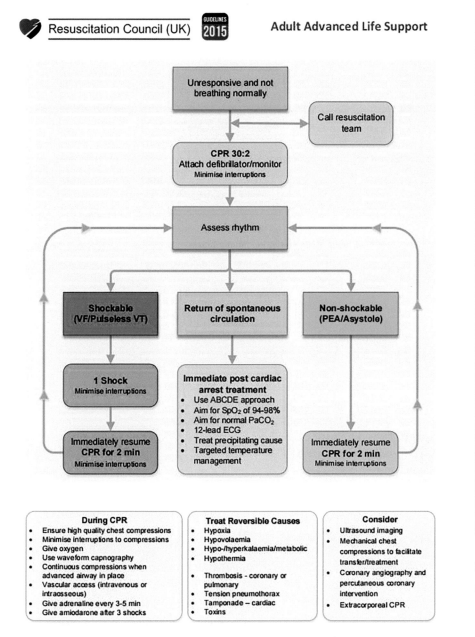

Key point

Treatment of VF/pulseless VT:

> As soon as a defibrillator arrives, apply the paddles or self-adhesive pads to the chest.

> Give one shock (150–200 J biphasic or 360 J monophasic).

> Do not reassess the rhythm or check for a pulse.

> Resume CPR for 2 minutes then reassess the ECG on the monitor.

> If VF is still present, give a second shock (150–200 J biphasic or 360 J monophasic).

> Resume CPR for 2 minutes then reassess the ECG on the monitor.

> If VF is still present, give 1 mg epinephrine (adrenaline) intravenously and then a third shock (150–200 J biphasic or 360 J monophasic).

> Resume CPR for 2 minutes then reassess the ECG on the monitor.

Fig 3 Resuscitation Council UK 2015 guidelines for ALS. (Reproduced with the kind permission of the Resuscitation Council (UK).) ALS, advanced life support; CPR, cardiopulmonary resuscitation; ECG, electrocardiogram; PEA, pulseless electrical activity; VF, ventricular fibrillation; VT, ventricular tachycardia.

Traditionally an endotracheal tube – a cuffed airway, placed within the trachea to enable both oxygenation and ventilation – was used to provide a definitive airway. The ease of placement of the laryngeal mask airway means that they are now more widely used, although they can potentially result in a higher risk of aspiration.

Categories of cardiac arrest

Two major categories are recognised: shockable (ventricular fibrillation (VF) or pulseless ventricular tachycardia (VT)); and non-shockable (previously subdivided into asystole and pulseless electrical activity).

Note the following:

> If a perfusing rhythm is present on reassessing the ECG on the monitor, try to palpate a pulse. Rhythm checks should be brief and pulse checks only performed if a perfusing rhythm is present.

> If an organised rhythm is present during a period of CPR, do not suspend the CPR unless the patient starts to show signs of life. If a perfusing rhythm has been restored, giving chest compressions does not increase the chances of VF recurring.

> If VF/VT persists after three shocks, give IV amiodarone 300 mg.

> Recommence CPR.

> Check electrode/paddle positions and contact.

> Obtain and secure the patient's airway and administer high-flow oxygen.

> Obtain intravenous access.

> Administer 1 mg epinephrine (adrenaline) intravenously every 3–5 minutes.

> Assess for potentially reversible causes.

> Reassess rhythm and defibrillate as necessary.

Epinephrine (adrenaline) is the first-line vasopressor, although it has not been shown to improve survival. Vasopressin is an alternative, but its use is not widespread.

Potentially reversible causes of non-VF/VT

> Hypoxia – ensure 100% oxygen is being administered, preferably via an endotracheal tube or laryngeal mask airway.

> Hypovolaemia – administer a rapid fluid bolus of 500–1,000 mL 0.9% saline; palpate for an abdominal aortic aneurysm; and check for rectal bleeding.

> Hypo-/hyperkalaemia and metabolic disorders – check the patient's clinical history (if available) for clues. If they have a known renal disease, presume hyperkalaemia is present and give 10 mL 10% calcium chloride or calcium gluconate IV.

> Hypothermia – the patient is never dead until they are warm and dead.

> Tension pneumothorax – consider especially in patients with pre-existing lung disease or who are on a ventilator. Look for asymmetrical chest, deviated trachea and unilateral absence of breath sounds. Immediate needle decompression of the affected side is mandatory.

> Tamponade – diagnosis is difficult: there is nothing to lose by attempting pericardiocentesis.

> Toxins – including drug overdose: check clinical history for clues.

> Thrombosis – always consider as a potential primary diagnosis or an MI.

Further comments

Antiarrhythmics in the management of cardiac arrest

There is no clear evidence for the use of antiarrhythmics in cardiac arrest. Although atropine is of use for haemodynamically significant bradycardia, its use in asystole is based on limited data. In cases of VF, amiodarone administered following three initial shocks has been shown to improve the short-term survival of patients until hospital admission, compared with placebo or lidocaine (lignocaine).

What role do buffers have in the management of cardiac arrest?

Adequate ventilation and tissue perfusion is the best way to treat the combined metabolic and respiratory acidosis seen in cardiac arrest. In the specific cases of arrest associated with tricyclic antidepressant overdose, hyperkalaemia and pre-existing metabolic acidosis, giving sodium bicarbonate intravenously may be of benefit. However a survival benefit has not been proven for cardiac arrest in general.

What role does pacing have in the management of cardiac arrest?

External pacing of asystole has shown no clinical benefit. Pacing may be of occasional use for the treatment of ventricular standstill.

Outcome following cardiac arrest

Return of spontaneous circulation (ROSC) occurs in about 30% of in-hospital cardiac arrests, but only around 15% of patients survive to hospital discharge. Only 2% of out-of-hospital arrests survive to hospital discharge. The survival rate for VF/VT is 10–15 times higher than for non-VF/VT. Survival from VF/VT correlates with the time taken before the first shock is applied, with approximately a 10% reduction in patient survival for each minute taken. Over 80% of successful resuscitations from VF/VT occur with one of the first three shocks.

If you are successful in resuscitating the patient, what should be done?

> Transfer them to an appropriate area for monitoring and treatment.

> Monitoring – ECG, SaO_2 and non-invasive BP.

> Treatment – high-flow oxygen.

> Debrief of the medical team and nursing staff involved (a nominated person is to complete a cardiac arrest audit form if it is standard hospital practice).

> Routine investigations – ECG, electrolytes, renal function, chest radiograph and arterial blood gases (ABGs).

> Other investigations – pursue reversible factors as dictated by clinical suspicion.

If the patient remains unconscious they will require transfer to the ICU if active management is to be pursued. Current European guidelines for management on the ICU recommend targeted temperature management with the aim of avoiding hyperthermia. Patients should be maintained at a temperature of 32–36°C for 24 hours and then prevented from achieving hyperthermia for a further 72 hours. Patients should also be managed to achieve normoxia, normocapnia and normoglycaemia.

When should an unsuccessful attempt at cardiopulmonary resuscitation be stopped?

If ROSC does not occur promptly, consideration must be given to termination of the attempt. Delays of more than 5 minutes before the start of BLS or more than 30 minutes to defibrillation are associated with a very poor prognosis. The presence of systemic sepsis, disseminated cancer and major organ failure are also predictors of very poor outcome. Age itself is not an independent predictor for the success of resuscitation, but comorbidities are more common and result in lower survival rates in older people. Hypothermia and the ingestion of some cerebral depressants (sedatives, hypnotics and narcotics) provide some measure of cerebral protection, but in the absence of reversible factors, attempts to resuscitate a patient from non-VF/VT arrest should be terminated after 20 minutes.

Should relatives be allowed to watch resuscitation attempts?

In many emergency departments and medical admission units it has become standard practice to allow relatives to observe resuscitation. The presence of family members during resuscitation efforts has been shown to aid the grieving process should resuscitation prove unsuccessful, but families should not be encouraged to enter the resuscitation room if they are reluctant.

Hazard

Relatives should only be allowed to observe resuscitation if there is a trained member of staff present whose sole responsibility is to support them; to have relatives watching with no one to explain what is going on and attend to their needs is asking for trouble.

1.3.2 Chest pain and hypotension

Case history

A 48-year-old male taxi driver has been brought into the emergency department. He is complaining of chest pain and breathlessness. He has a pulse rate of 130 beats per minute and his BP is 80/40mm Hg. You are asked to see him urgently by the nurse in charge.

Introduction

Key point

In dealing with a patient who is very ill, resuscitation should begin immediately and history taking, examination and investigation should be concurrent. Starting to take a detailed history from someone who is dying is likely to end in death rather than good medicine!

The priorities are:

> Resuscitate – airway, breathing and circulation (ABC).

> Try and establish a diagnosis (Table 5).

Resuscitation

Regardless of the specific diagnosis, your priorities must be to correct any problem with airway, breathing or circulation.

Key point

Get help early for any patient who is extremely unwell. Don't worry about establishing a diagnosis – ask for senior assistance. If necessary, put out a cardiac arrest call – it is much better to get the arrest team there to help than to wait until the patient's heart has stopped.

Table 5 Differential diagnosis of hypotensive collapse		
Common	**Must consider**	**Other causes**
Cardiovascular catastrophe: myocardial infarction, pulmonary embolism	Aortic dissection	Addisonian crisis
Hypovolaemia – particularly gastrointestinal blood loss	Tension pneumothorax	Hypothermia or hypothyroidism
A surgical cause – ruptured abdominal aortic aneurysm or a perforated viscus	Fluid loss from other causes, eg profound diarrhoea in an older person living alone	Cardiac tamponade
Sepsis – pneumonia and septicaemia	Multiple problems – particularly in older people (eg acute viral infection, inadequate fluid intake and complicating myocardial infarction)	

Airway/breathing

Ensure the patient's airway is patent: consider the placement of a nasopharyngeal or oropharyngeal airway if their conscious level is depressed. Apply an oxygen saturation monitor. Give high-flow oxygen. If the patient does not respond promptly to this or is ventilating inadequately then they may require intubation and ventilation: call for anaesthetic assistance sooner rather than later.

Hazard

Hypoxia kills – hypercarbia merely intoxicates

Even patients with known COPD should receive high-flow oxygen if they are *in extremis*. The oxygen may buy you enough time to institute other treatments and can then be slowly weaned according to blood gas analysis.

Circulation

Two large (grey) Venflons should be inserted into the antecubital fossae. If you are confident that a patient is hypovolaemic (exceedingly unlikely in this case), then give intravenous fluids quickly to the hypotensive patient until the circulation is restored. In most cases 0.9% saline (normal saline) will be appropriate initially. If there is evidence of acute blood loss then blood should be transfused: an emergency cross match should be available within 20–30 minutes, however intravenous fluids (or O-negative blood) can be given in the interim if required.

Key point

Resuscitation should be swift! There is no merit in resuscitating more slowly than is possible.

Key point

Fluid resuscitation of the hypovolaemic patient:

> Give 0.5 L 0.9% saline as fast as possible.

> Recheck peripheral perfusion, pulse, BP and JVP.

> If they are still hypovolaemic, give further 0.5 L 0.9% saline as fast as possible.

> Repeat cycle until signs of hypovolaemia are corrected.

> For severe sepsis initial fluid resuscitation is likely to require 30 mL/kg.

> Monitor closely for fluid overload, especially in older people and those with a history of heart failure – monitor pulse oximetry, JVP and the chest for crackles.

Insert a urinary catheter to monitor fluid output. The urinary catheter is the poor man's central venous pressure (CVP) line: it gives a measure of organ perfusion – a urine output of >0.5 mL/kg/h suggests that renal perfusion is adequate.

For those with persistent hypovolaemic shock (resistant hypotension and/or lactate over 4 mmol/L despite fluid resuscitation) a central/femoral venous

cannula maybe required. Note that it is difficult to access the internal jugular or subclavian vein in a patient who is breathless and cannot lie flat, or who is hypovolaemic, and an iatrogenic pneumo- or haemothorax can be fatal (Fig 4). A femoral line is a safer option, albeit with increased risk of infection (see Section 3.1.2).

Hazard

A 'normal' CVP reading does not necessarily mean that the patient would not benefit from more fluid.

Right-sided cardiac pressures reveal only part of the picture – it is possible to have a normal or high right atrial pressure at a time when the left ventricular filling is inadequate, eg with major pulmonary embolus (PE) or right-sided heart failure. If in doubt, give a fluid bolus of 250 mL and observe the response carefully.

If the patient remains hypotensive when intravascular volume has been restored, consider:

> The need for an additional fluid challenge – but do not induce fluid overload and pulmonary oedema, which could occur in this scenario.

> Inotropes – these can be used if there is circulatory pump failure. Vasoconstricting drugs may be necessary if vasodilatation is a part of the pathological process, eg sepsis. However, before escalating treatment in this way, the appropriateness of intensive care for the individual patient must be discussed and ratified.

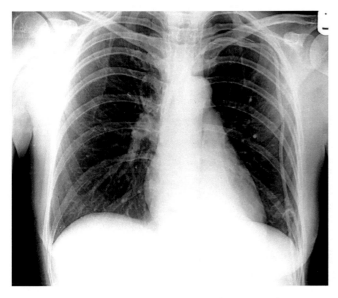

Fig 4 Left subclavian line, iatrogenic left pneumothorax.

Key point

When managing the hypotensive patient:

> Check airway and breathing.

> Give high-flow oxygen.

> Check if they are hypovolaemic; or is there another reason for their hypotension?

> If they are hypovolaemic give the correct fluid quickly.

> Is specific treatment indicated for the particular primary pathology?

> If they are still hypotensive – proceed to invasive haemodynamic measurement, inotropic and/or vasoconstricting drugs as indicated.

History of the presenting problem

Chest pain

> Dull, crushing central chest pain radiating to the neck or arms in association with nausea, vomiting, pallor and sweating would suggest a primary cardiac cause.

> The chest pain associated with PE may be dull, sharp or pleuritic.

> Sharp, tearing chest pain radiating to the back may indicate a dissecting aortic aneurysm.

> Could this be pain coming from an abdominal pathology?

Breathlessness

> Did the breathlessness come on suddenly or gradually? Sudden onset (in an instant) suggests pneumothorax, large airway obstruction or PE. Is there any suggestion that the patient has had multiple small PEs?

> Has the patient suffered from orthopnoea or paroxysmal nocturnal dyspnoea? These would suggest pulmonary oedema, but be aware that a patient with any cause of breathlessness will not want to lie down.

Any other features?

> Has the patient been feverish or systemically unwell? Could he have a severe pneumonia?

> Has the patient recently been immobile, got a history of cancer or been on a long flight? Leg pain, swelling or haemoptysis would clearly point towards PE in this context.

Other relevant history

It will clearly be important to find out if the patient has previously had problems with angina or MI, or (much less likely) any of the other diagnoses listed in Table 5. If he says 'the pain is just like when I had a heart attack last year', then the diagnosis is almost made.

Examination

Key point

When assessing any patient who presents acutely the first thing to do is to decide whether they are well, ill, very ill or nearly dead – it is vital for appropriate management to quickly decide which category they are in.

Overall assessment of the adequacy of the cardiovascular system

> If cardiac output is impaired, there is often a marked cut-off peripherally between warm, dry skin and a cold, clammy feel. Run your hand down the patient's arm, starting from the shoulder, and observe where the change occurs. Patients who are septic have a high cardiac output with low systemic resistance, such that they are peripherally vasodilated with warm, sweaty skin.

> Check the capillary return by pressing on the nailbed to blanch it and then measuring the time taken for the colour to return on releasing the pressure: normally it should be less than 2 seconds, more than 5 seconds is clearly abnormal.

> Heart rate, rhythm, lying and standing BP (or sitting, if the patient is too unwell to stand), and height of the JVP should always be measured to assess fluid status. A postural drop of >20 mmHg systolic and/or 10 mmHg diastolic points and/or an increase in pulse of >20 beats per minute points towards hypovolaemia. Measure the JVP in centimetres from the angle of Louis, angling the patient up or down until venous pulsation is seen – it is not good enough to settle for 'venous pressure not elevated'.

> Simple measures of organ perfusion include the ability of the patient to respond to questioning and the amount of urine produced per hour.

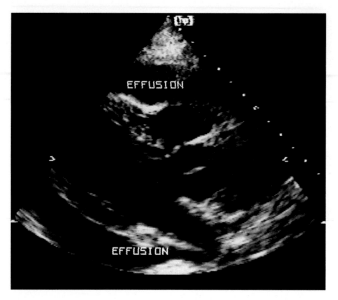

Fig 5 An echocardiogram of a large pericardial effusion.

Cardiovascular

In addition to assessing the overall adequacy of the cardiovascular system, check carefully for the following when performing the cardiovascular examination:

> Can you feel the left radial pulse as well as the right? If it seems to be diminished, measure BP in both arms and consider aortic dissection.

> Can you hear any murmurs? Acute mitral valve regurgitation or a ventricular septal defect (VSD) can complicate an acute MI (AMI) and cause catastrophic heart failure. Always consider the possibility of bacterial endocarditis when a murmur is discovered.

> Consider PE – look for leg swelling, elevated JVP, right ventricular heave, right ventricular gallop and loud P2.

> Consider pericardial effusion – it is easy to overlook this possibility (Fig 5), but the signs of pulsus paradoxus (an exaggeration of the normal fall in systolic BP that occurs on inspiration to >10 mmHg, which must be measured with a sphygmomanometer) and elevation of the venous pressure with inspiration (Kussmaul's sign) should be a part of your routine examination.

Respiratory

Key point

A tension pneumothorax can present with circulatory collapse or cardiac arrest, so look specifically for the following:

> The chest often looks asymmetrical, with the affected side 'blown up'.

> The trachea is deviated away from the affected side.

> The mediastinum is shifted away from the affected side, which can be detected by finding displacement of the apex beat or shift of the area of cardiac dullness on percussion.

> The affected side of the chest is silent.

In this case it would be much more likely that you would hear the crackles of pulmonary oedema, but look also for signs that might indicate pneumonic consolidation (dullness to percussion and bronchial breathing) or a pleural rub (consistent with PE or pneumonia).

Abdominal

A number of abdominal pathologies can cause collapse with or without chest pain. Check for abdominal distention, bruising in the flanks, aortic aneurysm (palpate deliberately in the epigastrium), herniae and peritonism. Consider the following diagnoses: ruptured abdominal aortic aneurysm, perforated viscus/spleen, pancreatitis, cholecystitis/cholangitis and intestinal obstruction.

Hazard

Coma and hypotension: which came first, the chicken or the egg?

If a patient who is unconscious is also hypotensive, it is far more likely that the hypotension is the cause of the unconsciousness than vice versa. Primary intracerebral pathologies that result in hypotension are rare; hypotension causing inadequate cerebral perfusion is common.

Investigation

Tests to be requested immediately in the emergency department are:

> Pulse oximetry; finger-prick blood glucose.

> ECG – looking in particular at rate/ rhythm (is the pulse of 130 beats per minute sinus rhythm, or an arrhythmia that might benefit from treatment?) and for evidence of MI.

> Routine blood tests – FBC, electrolytes, renal/liver/bone profile, C-reactive protein (CRP), clotting, troponin and D-dimer if possible DVT/PE.

> Cultures – blood, urine. Sputum and cerebrospinal fluid (CSF) as indicated.

> Arterial blood gases (ABGs) – pulse oximetry can be unreliable in patients who are hypotensive. Measurement of their ABGs is essential to check oxygen levels and pH.

> Chest radiograph – this may give vital information. A widened mediastinum or evidence of air under the diaphragm may reveal the diagnosis.

> Other investigations – as determined by clinical suspicion, eg a CT angiogram for aortic dissection or CT pulmonary angiogram for PE.

Management

In addition to resuscitation described above, also consider the following.

Antibiotics

If there is a possibility of sepsis as a diagnosis, then prescribe broad-spectrum antibiotics. The choice will depend on the likely source, the local prevalence of organisms, recent travel and previous antibiotic exposure. Involve the microbiologist as

early as possible. Remember that sepsis can present atypically and always take blood cultures before prescribing antibiotics.

Other specific conditions

Any of the conditions listed in Table 5 will require rapid specific treatment:

> MI – clearly the most likely diagnosis in this case (see Section 1.3.3)

> PE – see Section 1.3.8

> tension pneumothorax – see Section 1.3.12

> gastrointestinal haemorrhage – see Section 1.3.13

> intra-abdominal catastrophe – arrange for urgent surgical consultation if the main problem seems to be abdominal.

1.3.3 Acute coronary syndrome

Case history
A 57-year-old businessman presents to the emergency department with a history of severe central crushing chest pain of 1 hour's duration. This followed a stressful business meeting. The nurse in charge asks you whether he should be transferred for primary percutaneous coronary intervention (PCI).

Introduction

Hazard
Between 2% and 4% of patients with an acute myocardial infarction (AMI) are discharged inappropriately from the emergency department. This is more likely to occur in women than men, and also in older people and non-Caucasians.

The most likely diagnosis is acute coronary syndrome (ACS) – immediate priorities are:

Resuscitation and immediate assessment

> Airway, breathing and circulation (ABC).

> Administer high-flow oxygen and apply a saturation monitor.

> Check the heart rate and rhythm. Feel for pulses and check the BP in both arms. Check peripheral perfusion (see Section 1.3.2). Get intravenous access.

> All patients with a possible ACS should have continuous cardiac monitoring because cardiac arrhythmias are common in this condition and need prompt treatment.

Diagnosis

> Look carefully at the ECG – if it is diagnostic for ST elevation acute myocardial infarction (STEMI) then consider transferring for immediate reperfusion therapy.

Key point
The ECG criteria for STEMI are:

> 1 mm or more ST-segment elevation in two contiguous limb leads

> 2 mm or more ST-segment elevation in two contiguous chest leads

> new left bundle branch block.

History of the presenting problem

Look for features in the history to suggest that this patient is suffering from an ACS:

> Patients with more severe pain are more likely to have an ACS, but be wary – social, professional and age-related differences influence the presentation of symptoms. Women are more likely to complain of referred pain to the neck, jaw and back.

> Ischaemic pain is more likely to be diffuse and of longer duration. The pain of an acute myocardial infarction (AMI) is likely to be described as a constant pressure and may be associated with sweating, nausea and vomiting.

Other relevant history

The National Institute for Health and Care Excellence (NICE) guidelines suggest that the risk of myocardial ischaemia is assessed according to the following features:

> Nature of symptoms – pain in chest, arms, back or jaw lasting longer than 15 minutes; associated symptoms, including nausea and vomiting, sweating and breathlessness; chest pain associated with haemodynamic instability; new onset chest pain or deterioration in previously stable angina.

> Presence of cardiovascular risk factors – smoking, hypertension, hypercholesterolaemia, diabetes, obesity, family history.

> Presence of known ischaemic heart disease (or symptoms that are strongly suggestive of this) and any previous treatment, as well as the results of previous investigations for chest pain.

Examination

Attention will clearly focus on cardiac and respiratory examination, but look for the following features that would suggest a diagnosis of ACS:

> The patient with ischaemic pain is likely to have autonomic signs – they may be sweating, clammy, cool and pale.

> AMI is more likely if the patient has hypotension and a third heart sound.

> Exclusion of other diagnoses – check peripheral pulses to rule out aortic dissection; listen for murmurs and pericardial or pleural rubs.

Investigation

Electrocardiogram

This is clearly the most important initial investigation in this case: look carefully for any signs of STEMI (Fig 6) and act immediately. Around one-third of patients with an AMI will not have ST elevation on arrival – look for ST depression, T-wave inversion, Q-waves or any conduction defect. If the ECG is normal on arrival and the clinical suspicion is high, then arrange for serial ECGs.

Look also for features of pericarditis. Typical ECG changes are of peaked T-waves and ST-segments which are elevated and concave upwards. Another ECG change suggestive of acute pericarditis is depression of the PR interval (Fig 7).

Blood tests

Troponin(s), electrolytes, renal and liver function tests, blood sugar, lipid levels, FBC and clotting.

Chest radiograph

Measure heart size, exclude pulmonary oedema, and look for the widened mediastinum of aortic dissection.

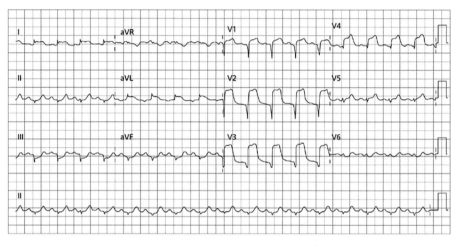

Fig 6 An ECG of acute anterior myocardial infarction (MI) with early Q-wave formation.

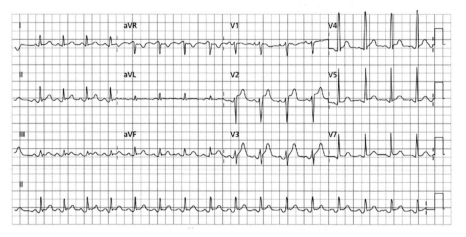

Fig 7 An ECG of acute pericarditis – the ST-segment changes are obvious, but note also the depressed PR interval shown especially in leads II and augmented vector foot (aVF).

Management – ST elevation myocardial infarction

General

> Administer oxygen if required, start cardiac monitoring and offer pain relief with opioids.

> Aspirin 300 mg if not already given.

> Assess for complications such as left ventricular failure and tachyarrhythmias.

Reperfusion therapy

Immediately assess eligibility for coronary reperfusion therapy (either primary percutaneous coronary intervention (PCI) or thrombolysis).

Primary percutaneous coronary intervention

Primary PCI is the preferred reperfusion strategy for STEMI in patients presenting within 12 hours of symptoms (as long as this will not take more than 2 hours longer than it would take to give thrombolysis).

> Activate primary PCI pathway and transfer to primary PCI centre immediately. Target door-to-balloon time is 90 minutes.

> Give additional antiplatelet: clopidogrel, prasugrel or ticagrelor.

> At time of PCI give bivalirudin if previously treated with clopidogrel. If previously treated with prasugrel or ticagrelor then give heparin (unfractionated or low molecular weight).

Thrombolysis

Offer thrombolysis if presenting within 12 hours of symptoms, primary PCI cannot be delivered within 120 minutes of when thrombolysis could be given, and there are no contraindications.

> Thrombolysis should be started within 30 minutes of presentation.

> When giving thrombolysis give an antithrombin at the same time.

> Patients with contraindications to thrombolysis (see below) should be transferred for PCI even if this cannot occur within 90 minutes.

> Repeat ECG 60–90 minutes after thrombolysis. If this shows residual ST-segment elevation then offer immediate angiography with PCI if indicated.

Key point

Contraindications to thrombolysis:

> any previous history of haemorrhagic stroke

> structural cerebrovascular lesions, including neoplasms

> ischaemic stroke within previous 6 months

> major surgery, trauma or bleeding within the preceding 2 weeks

> BP >200/110 mmHg

> suspected aortic dissection

> known bleeding disorder

> gastrointestinal (GI) bleeding within last month.

Management – unstable angina / non-ST elevation myocardial infarction

General

> Administer oxygen if required, start cardiac monitoring and offer pain relief with opioids.

> Sublingual nitrates, and consider intravenous or buccal nitrates if pain recurs.

> Assess for complications such as left ventricular failure and tachyarrhythmias.

Antiplatelet therapy

> Aspirin 300 mg if not already given and then commence 75 mg daily.

> Clopidogrel 300 mg loading dose, followed by 75 mg daily for up to 12 months.

> Consider glycoprotein IIb/IIIa inhibitors (eg tirofiban) in patients at intermediate–high risk of adverse cardiovascular events (see below) and those in whom PCI is planned.

Antithrombin therapy

> Offer fondaparinux unless coronary angiography is planned within 24 hours (if angiography is planned then use unfractionated heparin as an alternative.)

Coronary angiography

> Patients at intermediate or high risk should be offered coronary angiography within 96 hours of admission.

> Consider ischaemia testing prior to discharge in patients who have not had coronary angiography.

Risk stratification

> NICE recommends assessment of the risk of future adverse cardiovascular events to estimate 6-month mortality eg Global Registry of Acute Cardiac Events (GRACE). Predicted 6-month mortality below 3% is viewed as low risk, 3–6% is intermediate, and above 6% high risk.

> Another popular risk stratification system is the thrombolysis in myocardial infarction (TIMI) score, which predicts the risk of all-cause mortality, new or recurrent MI, or severe ischaemia requiring urgent revascularisation at 14 days.

Key point

TIMI risk score

This is determined as follows:

Risk factors	Points
Age >65 years	1
More than three coronary artery disease (CAD) risk factors (family history, hypertension, hypercholesterolaemia, diabetes mellitus and smoking)	1
Known coronary artery disease (stenosis >50%)	1
Aspirin use in the past 7 days	1
Presentation points	
Recent severe angina (<24 hours)	1
Raised cardiac markers	1
ST-segment change >0.5 mm	1

Risk score = total points (0–7); HIGH RISK = score >3

Secondary prevention and rehabilitation

All patients who have had an MI should receive treatment with the following drugs unless contraindicated:

> Dual antiplatelet therapy – aspirin should be continued indefinitely, with a second antiplatelet agent given for up to 12 months.

> Statins – measure lipids on admission and start atorvastatin 80 mg daily.

> Angiotensin-converting enzyme (ACE) inhibitor – should be started when the patient is haemodynamically stable.

> Beta-blocker – should be started as soon as possible unless contraindicated, and up-titrated as tolerated. Continue for at least 12 months and indefinitely if there is left ventricular (LV) dysfunction. Consider diltiazem if beta-blockade is contraindicated, but avoid dihydropyridine calcium channel blockers (eg nifedipine).

Patients should also be offered:

> Assessment of left ventricular function – echocardiography can identify regional wall abnormalities in patients with cardiac ischaemia and may also pick up important prognostic information such as systolic dysfunction.

> Lifestyle advice including smoking cessation, diet and weight management and exercise.

> Cardiac rehabilitation.

Further comments

Oxygen therapy in ACS

International guidelines differ over whether all patients with an acute MI (AMI) should be treated with oxygen. Current NICE guidelines for assessment of patients with chest pain recommend only giving oxygen to those patients who require supplemental oxygen to achieve their target saturations. British Thoracic Society (BTS) guidelines also state that oxygen is not required unless the patient is hypoxaemic and to achieve oxygen saturations of 94–98%, or 88–92% if the patient is at risk of hypercapnia.

Hyperglycaemia in acute STEMI

Early trials suggested that tight glucose control using intravenous insulin was beneficial in AMI (DIGAMI trial), but this has not been confirmed in subsequent trials. The European Society of Cardiology guidelines recommend managing hyperglycaemia to maintain a blood sugar concentration <11 mmol/L but avoiding hypoglycaemia. This may require a variable rate insulin infusion.

Aortic dissection

If dissection is suspected, the definitive investigations are either CT (Fig 8) or transoesophageal echocardiography (Fig 9). Surgery should be considered urgently for patients with proximal aortic dissection.

Pericarditis

A therapeutic trial of aspirin or other non-steroidal anti-inflammatory drugs (NSAIDs) can sometimes help in diagnosing pericarditis; relief of pericarditic pain commonly occurs within 20 minutes.

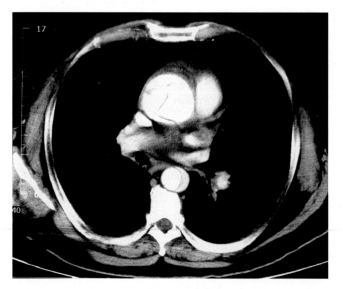

Fig 8 A mediastinal CT scan showing the classical appearances of aortic dissection: note the 'tennis-ball' appearance in the ascending and descending aorta.

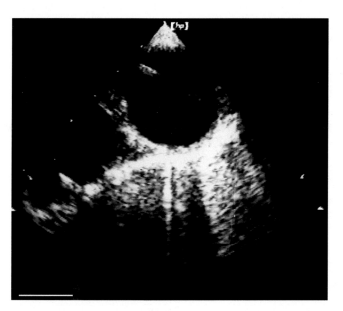

Fig 9 Transoesophageal echocardiogram showing the flap of dissection in the aorta.

Oesophageal pain
Inevitably, there will be some situations in which it is impossible to decide between an oesophageal and a cardiac aetiology. In these situations, your fallback position must be to 'consider it cardiac until proved otherwise'.

Key point
Diagnostic uncertainty
If you do not know the diagnosis, be honest with yourself and with the patient. It does not mean that you have 'failed': the diagnosis may be impossible to make. Consider the major diagnoses discussed. Therapeutic trials may give aid diagnostically, but the default position must be to consider the most serious potential conditions and treat them appropriately until further evidence has secured the diagnosis.

1.3.4 Hypotension in acute coronary syndrome

Case history
A 72-year-old man is admitted to the coronary care unit with chest pain. He has known ischaemic heart disease and has had previous coronary artery bypass grafts. On presentation he was sweaty, with BP 120/70 mmHg and a clear chest. His ECG on arrival in the emergency department showed ST-segment depression and T-wave changes inferiorly. He was commenced on maximal medical therapy, including aspirin, IV nitrates, IV beta-blockers, low-molecular-weight heparin and clopidogrel.

It is now 6 hours since his admission: he has become drowsy and his BP has fallen to 70/50 mmHg. You are bleeped to review him urgently.

Introduction
The cause of profound hypotension in a patient with an ACS can usually be established by examining the patient, obtaining an ECG and chest radiograph, and review of the drug chart.

Key point
Check airway, breathing and circulation, and begin management immediately:

> Administer high-flow oxygen and monitor pulse oximetry.
> Check heart rate and rhythm, and the BP in both arms.
> Obtain intravenous access (if not already established).
> Give 250 mL fluid bolus if the chest is clear.
> Stop any drugs that may be contributing to hypotension.
> Call for help early.

History of presenting problem
This man is unlikely to respond well to attempts to take a lengthy history from him, but important things to find out from him and from scrutiny of the observation charts are:

> Is he in pain? Ongoing or new pain in an ACS may indicate development of STEMI – an AMI – or cardiac rupture.

> Has his BP fallen suddenly or gradually? A sudden onset of low BP in association with new chest pain is again suggestive of cardiac rupture. Low BP in association with breathlessness resulting from left ventricular pump failure tends to be more gradual in onset.

> What drugs has he been given? Look closely for a temporal relationship between his hypotension and the administration of drugs. Intravenous nitrates and morphine are likely to cause his BP to drop.

Examination

Key features to concentrate on are:

> Peripheral perfusion – it is a poor prognostic sign if the patient is shut down; how far up the arms and legs are they cold?

> Heart rate and rhythm – could a secondary tachycardia or bradycardia be the cause of hypotension?

> BP in both arms – could the patient have had an aortic dissection in association with an inferior MI?

> JVP – if this is markedly raised, then consider right ventricular infarction, VSD, tamponade or pulmonary embolism (PE). A low JVP would be a surprise in this clinical context, but if found consider the possibility of gastrointestinal bleeding – especially if thrombolysis has been given.

> Auscultation of the heart – a new pansystolic murmur would suggest a VSD or mitral regurgitation as a result of chordal or papillary muscle rupture; a gallop rhythm would be expected.

> Crackles in the chest, indicating pulmonary oedema.

> Pulse oximetry.

Quantitate the patient's 'drowsiness' by checking his Glasgow Coma Scale (GCS) score. Depression of consciousness may be due to hypotension, opioids (how much morphine has he had? Are the pupils pinpoint? If so, give naloxone).

Investigation

See Sections 1.3.3 and 1.3.4 for fuller discussion, but the following are clearly vital in this case:

> ECG – repeat to assess cardiac rhythm and look for evidence of ongoing ischaemia. In particular, has an inferior infarct pattern developed and are there signs of right ventricular infarction?

> Chest radiograph – will give some information about pre-existing chest and cardiac conditions (cardiac shape and size) as well as an assessment of pulmonary congestion.

> Echocardiogram – likely to be the most useful investigation in this case. In particular, in detecting acute mitral regurgitation, VSD and tamponade; and also in enabling assessment of global overall right and left ventricular function and focal abnormalities thereof.

Management

Again see Sections 1.3.3 and 1.3.4 for fuller discussion, but note the following particularly relevant to this case:

Key point

Has anyone spoken to the relatives and informed them of what has happened? This man is desperately ill and may die soon.

General supportive measures

> High-flow oxygen and respiratory support with the aim of maximising oxygen delivery. Use of continuous positive airway pressure (CPAP) may decrease intubation rates, but no decease on mortality has yet been shown. Consider intubation if there is acute respiratory failure which is not responding to medical treatment.

> Analgesia – if the patient is in pain do not withhold adequate analgesia, but give small doses at a time (eg morphine 2.5 mg IV, with antiemetic).

> Fluids – the hypotensive, hypoxic patient with bilateral crackles will not respond well to a fluid challenge; but give a cautious fluid bolus (250 mL) if they are hypotensive with a clear chest, even if they have a raised JVP.

In the setting of an inferior MI this could reflect right ventricular ischaemia and volume loading alone may improve the cardiac output.

> Monitoring – haemodynamically unstable patients need close monitoring. CVP lines have a role, but be cautious with the readings, watch the trend and do not over interpret. Do not underestimate the value of a urinary catheter and measurement of hourly urine output in assessment of the circulation.

Other methods of circulatory support

> Inotropes – evidence for their benefit is limited. They can obviously raise the arterial pressure, which looks better on the observation charts, but there is no compelling evidence that they improve prognosis. The resulting high systemic vascular resistance means they should be used with caution and for a limited time only because they can lead to a further decrease in end-organ tissue perfusion.

> Intra-aortic balloon counterpulsation – another holding method whose use should be restricted to patients with an underlying condition that can be treated (percutaneous coronary intervention (PCI), valve replacement, repair of VSD or – not appropriate in this case – heart transplant) or that will recover spontaneously (early post AMI, post surgery or myocarditis).

Specific measures

Specialist advice is needed: would this man benefit from PCI, valve replacement or repair of VSD?

Key point

If there are no obvious reversible or treatable factors and no satisfactory response to initial medical treatment, then palliation of symptoms must be the priority.

1.3.5 Tachyarrhythmia

Case history

You are called to the medical assessment unit to assess a 72-year-old woman with palpitations who is complaining of chest pain. The nurse looking after her is worried that she has a heart rate of 150 beats per minute and is hypotensive.

Introduction

Some arrhythmias left untreated can cause cardiac arrest, while others may need no immediate treatment. You need to be able to recognise common arrhythmias in order to know which need immediate treatment.

Key point

The adverse features of tachyarrhythmias are:

> shock (systolic BP <90 mmHg)
> myocardial ischaemia
> heart failure
> syncope.

Key point

Management of a tachyarrhythmia associated with adverse features should include the following:

> Call for help immediately.
> Assess using the airway, breathing, circulation (ABC) approach.
> Give the patient high-flow oxygen.
> Insert intravenous access.
> Place them on a cardiac monitor – monitor BP and oxygen saturations.
> Record 12-lead ECG.
> Prepare for synchronised cardioversion immediately, with sedation or a general anaesthetic.

History of the presenting problem

The risks of coronary artery disease and myocardial ischaemia increase with age. Ventricular tachycardia (VT) is far more likely in someone who has known coronary artery disease or has had a previous AMI. Ask about previous episodes of palpitations and episodes of syncope. Establish whether the patient is symptomatic: Do they have chest pain (as this woman does)? Are they breathless? Do they feel dizzy or faint?

In young patients with no history of ischaemic heart disease ask about previous syncope or palpitations. You should also specifically ask about family history of cardiac problems, including sudden cardiac death or relatives who have died suddenly at a young age (syncope and sudden cardiac death may have been misdiagnosed as epilepsy).

Other relevant history

Get the old notes: old ECGs are invaluable. Is there evidence of an innate electrical abnormality, eg classical accessory pathways of the Wolff–Parkinson–White (WPW) or the Lown–Ganong–Levine syndromes? Look for an echocardiogram result: what is the left ventricular function; and is there evidence of structural heart problems, eg valve disease or cardiomyopathy? Any of these increase the likelihood of a serious arrhythmia.

Examination

An overall assessment of the adequacy of the cardiovascular system is required, as described in Section 1.3.2. If the arrhythmia is not well tolerated the heart may start to fail as cardiac output falls; and if there is inadequate time in diastole for cardiac filling the myocardium becomes ischaemic, which will be worse if there is underlying coronary artery disease. These clinical features will dictate the speed at which treatment is needed.

Investigation

After checking for clinical features that would indicate adverse prognosis, get a 12-lead ECG immediately.

Is this a broad or narrow complex tachycardia?

Are the QRS complexes narrow (<120 ms) or broad (>120 ms)? Broad complex tachycardias tend to be less well tolerated because there is often underlying heart disease. If in doubt, always assume a broad complex tachycardia is a VT until proved otherwise: the use of verapamil to treat VT could cause severe and prolonged hypotension or even cardiac arrest; by contrast, attempts to correct a VT are unlikely to cause any further compromise in an supraventricular tachycardia (SVT).

Key point

Assume a broad complex tachycardia is a VT until proved otherwise.

Is a broad complex tachycardia a ventricular tachycardia or a supraventricular tachycardia with aberrant conduction?

Ventricular tachycardia (VT) is more likely if there is/are:

> atrioventricular (AV) dissociation – more QRS complexes than P-waves is diagnostic of VT

> very wide QRS complexes – the wider the complexes, the more likely that the origin of the arrhythmia is ventricular (Fig 10); QRS complexes >0.14 seconds wide are almost certain to be due to VT

> capture beats and fusion beats

> concordance – meaning that the QRS complexes have the same morphology across all the chest leads

> extreme left axis deviation or a change in axis from an old ECG.

An irregular broad complex tachycardia could be atrial fibrillation (AF) with bundle branch block or, less commonly, AF with ventricular pre-excitation. Polymorphic VT (torsades de pointes) is another possibility, but remember that this is unusual without any adverse features.

Regular narrow complex tachycardias:

> sinus tachycardia

> AV nodal re-entry tachycardia – the commonest type of SVT

> AV re-entrant tachycardia – pre-excitation including WPW syndrome

> atrial flutter with regular AV conduction; the most common block is 2:1, but others such as 4:1 are possible (see Fig 11).

Irregular narrow complex tachycardias:

> AF with an uncontrolled ventricular response (Fig 12).

> Atrial flutter with irregular AV conduction (variable block and hence irregular).

Other investigations

> Electrolytes – hypokalaemia, hypomagnesaemia and acidosis can precipitate arrhythmias.

> FBC – anaemia will exacerbate myocardial ischaemia.

> TSH as AF is a common complication of hyperthyroidism.

> Chest radiograph – heart size and pulmonary oedema.

> Echocardiogram – left ventricular function and other anatomical abnormality.

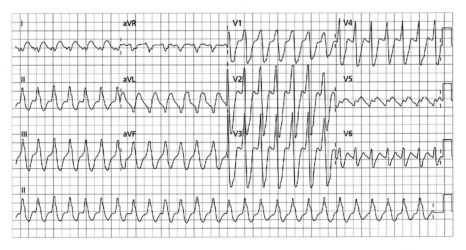

Fig 10 Ventricular tachycardia showing wide QRS complexes and concordance.

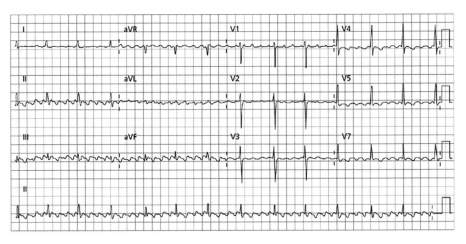

Fig 11 Atrial flutter with 4:1 AV block.

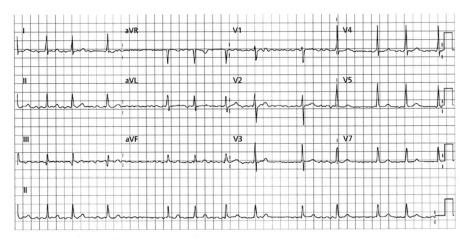

Fig 12 Atrial fibrillation.

Management

Tachycardia leading to haemodynamic compromise (unstable patients)

Synchronised direct-current (DC) cardioversion is required. Energy levels required depend on the underlying rhythm and the type of defibrillator (biphasic or monophasic). Ensure that the defibrillator is set to synchronised mode. Start with the following energy levels and increase incrementally if unsuccessful:

> atrial flutter or SVT – 50–75 J biphasic (100 J monophasic)

> AF or VT – 100 J biphasic (200 J monophasic).

If cardioversion is unsuccessful you can try moving the paddles to the anterior/posterior position with one paddle over the heart apex and the other below the right scapula to the right of the spine.

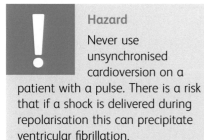

Hazard

Never use unsynchronised cardioversion on a patient with a pulse. There is a risk that if a shock is delivered during repolarisation this can precipitate ventricular fibrillation.

Tachycardia without haemodynamic compromise (stable patients)

Management will depend on the underlying rhythm.

Sinus tachycardia

Sinus tachycardia is a physiological response to stress. Management should be directed at the underlying cause: attempts to slow the heart rate by any other means will almost certainly do harm rather than good.

Supraventricular tachycardia

Vagal manoeuvres or adenosine are the treatments of choice.

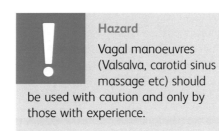

Hazard

Vagal manoeuvres (Valsalva, carotid sinus massage etc) should be used with caution and only by those with experience.

Adenosine is a naturally occurring purine nucleoside that is highly efficient at blocking the AV node. Its action lasts for seconds only, and it is not negatively inotropic. It is highly effective at terminating paroxysmal SVT with re-entrant circuits that include the AV node (AV re-entrant tachycardia and AV nodal re-entrant tachycardia). In other narrow-complex tachycardias (eg atrial flutter) it will reveal the underlying atrial rhythm by slowing the ventricular response.

Key point

Adenosine should be administered as follows:

> Ensure that you have continuous cardiac monitoring and ideally print the trace, starting when adenosine is given (this is helpful if diagnosis is in doubt).

> Start with a rapid intravenous bolus of 6 mg.

> Follow with up to two doses of 12 mg at intervals of 1–2 minutes.

> Each bolus should be given into a large vein followed immediately by a flush of saline.

Hazard

Adenosine is contraindicated in patients with/taking:

> asthma

> high-degree AV block (second- or third-degree heart block)

> dipyridamole – this drug potentiates the effect of adenosine.

If adenosine is contraindicated or fails to terminate a regular narrow-complex tachycardia without demonstrating that it is atrial flutter, then give a calcium channel blocker (verapamil or diltiazem). Beta-blockade is a reasonable alternative.

Atrial fibrillation

Recent onset (<48 hours) In haemodynamically stable patients where AF is known to be of recent onset (<48 hours) and not precipitated by intercurrent illness, the patient should undergo electrical cardioversion. Pharmacological cardioversion can be attempted if that fails. Amiodarone is both antiarrhythmic and rate limiting (see below for dosing regimen). Long-term anticoagulation treatment is not required if sinus rhythm is restored and a patient is thought to be at low risk of recurrence of AF.

Onset >48 hours ago If AF has been present for >48 hours and was not precipitated by intercurrent illness, the priority – after antithrombotic treatment – is rate control with a beta-blocker or a rate-limiting calcium channel blocker (eg diltiazem). Digoxin as monotherapy is only recommended in sedentary patients, but can be beneficial in patients with left ventricular dysfunction.

Elective cardioversion at 6 weeks can be considered if symptoms persist despite adequate rate control.

Anticoagulation

Patients with AF are at risk of stroke and the risks and benefits of anticoagulation need to be considered. NICE guidelines recommend that risk of stroke is assessed using the $CHA_2DS_2\text{-}VASc$ score (below). Risk of bleeding should also be taken into account. Anticoagulation, where indicated, can be with warfarin or with one of the novel anticoagulant drugs (apixaban, dabigatran or rivaroxaban).

Pill in the pocket

In patients with infrequent paroxysms of AF a 'pill-in-the-pocket' strategy can be useful if patients are aware of symptoms and when to take the drug. Flecainide can be used if there is no ischaemic or structural heart disease.

Hazard

If a patient in AF has WPW syndrome, then AV-node blocking drugs (including digoxin) should be avoided. Flecainide is an alternative, but not in the presence of left ventricle dysfunction. Call for specialist advice rather than 'having a go'.

Regular broad complex tachycardia

In the absence of adverse features, give amiodarone 300 mg intravenously over 20–60 minutes followed by 900 mg in the next 24 hours. Class Ic drugs should be avoided. Monitor the patient closely. If adverse features develop, be prepared to use electrical cardioversion.

Patients with polymorphic VT (torsades de pointes) should be treated with intravenous magnesium (8 mmol over 10 minutes). Other electrolyte disorders (especially hypokalaemia) should be corrected.

An algorithm to help in the diagnosis of broad complex tachycardia is shown in Fig 13.

Irregular broad complex tachycardia

Be cautious in the management of an irregular broad complex tachycardia. If it is AF with bundle branch block, treat as for AF (see above). If pre-excitation is present, then adenosine, digoxin and verapamil should be avoided; these drugs block the AV node and may increase accessory pathway conduction with the inherent danger of precipitating ventricular fibrillation (VF).

Key point

In the haemodynamically stable patient, give one antiarrhythmic agent. If this is unsuccessful in restoring normal rhythm, it will be safer to move to DC cardioversion rather than administering additional antiarrhythmic drugs.

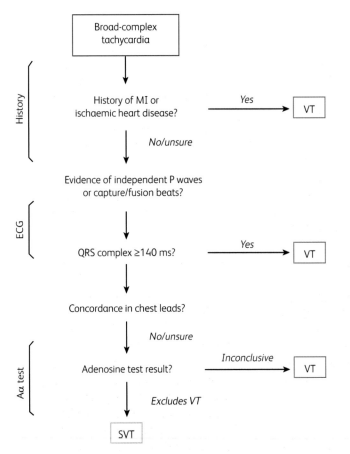

Fig 13 Algorithm to help decision making in broad complex tachycardia. ECG, electrocardiogram; MI, myocardial infarction; SVT, supraventricular tachycardia; VT, ventricular tachycardia.

1.3.6 Bradyarrhythmia

Case history

A 76-year-old woman is brought to the emergency department by ambulance having been found collapsed in her kitchen at home by her son when he went round to visit in the morning. She is normally independent and lives alone. She has a past medical history of hypertension, osteoarthritis and non-insulin dependent diabetes mellitus. You are called to review her urgently by the triage nurse, who finds her pulse rate to be 30 beats per minute.

Introduction

The first priority will be to check her other vital signs and make a judgment as to whether she is well enough to give a useful history. She may be tolerating her bradycardia well and be able to give an account of what has happened to her, but if she is not then you should immediately proceed from a rapid screening examination (head-to-toe screen and GCS / Abbreviated Mental Test scores (as appropriate)) to treatment.

The most obvious diagnosis from the details given is that the woman has developed complete heart block, but do not jump to conclusions – if she had a simple trip in the evening but hurt herself such that she could not get off the floor, then she may have a bradycardia due to hypothermia in the morning.

History of the presenting problem

If the patient is well enough to give a history, then pursue an account of the collapse itself. What details (if any) can she (or her son) remember? Try to get a precise account: 'What exactly were you doing … and then what happened … and then?' and note in particular the following:

> Did she get any warning? Absence of warning symptoms would be typical of cardiac syncope (Stokes–Adams attack).

> How long did it last? In most cases of cardiac syncope the period of unconsciousness usually lasts between 10–30 seconds.

> Did she injure herself when she collapsed?

> How did the son find her? Is there any evidence that she may have spent the night on the floor? Was she fully clothed when found, and what was the ambient temperature of her surroundings? If she spent the night on the floor, then it means that following the collapse she was not able to mobilise sufficiently to call for help or return to bed, which may have important implications in relation to the cause of the collapse. Also, spending the night on the floor will increase her risk of developing hypothermia, pressure sores and other associated injuries.

Other relevant history

Has she had previous similar events – syncope or presyncope? Is there any history of epilepsy, or any features to suggest that she could have had an unwitnessed fit (although this does not seem likely in this case)?

What medication is she on, and have any drugs been started recently? Enquire specifically about antihypertensives (especially beta-blockers), but also hypoglycaemic agents, analgesics, sedatives and anti-Parkinsonian medications, all of which can cause confusion and/or disturbance of consciousness.

Examination

If the woman is very unwell proceed as described in Sections 1.3.1 and 1.3.2, but otherwise concentrate on:

> What is she wearing? This may have some relevance as to at what time the collapse occurred.

> Signs of injury – in particular look at the pressure areas for signs that she has been immobile for a period; and consider specifically 'has she got a fractured hip?' by looking for a short, externally rotated leg.

> Temperature – is she hypothermic? Use a low-reading thermometer and take a rectal temperature.

> Cardiovascular – check heart rate and rhythm, peripheral perfusion and BP. Automated machines may give unreliable results in a patient with low cardiac output due to bradycardia, so check a manual BP reading.

> Respiratory – are there signs to suggest aspiration/hypostatic pneumonia?

> Neurological – assess her GCS score; also look for focal signs that might indicate she has had a stroke (most commonly dysphasia, hemianopia, facial asymmetry and hemiparesis).

> Signs to suggest hypothyroidism – general appearance and slow-relaxing tendon jerks.

Hazard

Do not forget hypothermia as a cause of profound bradycardia, especially in older people.

Investigation

Electrocardiogram

Is there heart block and, if so, is it first-, second- or third degree in type? (See Fig 14.) Generally speaking, the higher the degree of heart block, the less stable the situation. But this is by no means always the case and the decision on management should not be taken on the basis of the ECG alone. Alternatively, there may be AF with a slow ventricular response or even profound sinus bradycardia. Is there any indication of recent MI that might demand specific treatment?

Routine blood tests

Electrolytes, renal/liver/bone profile, glucose, creatine kinase (CK), troponin I/T and thyroid function tests. A very high CK (>10,000 IU/L – normal range (females) 24–170) with hypocalcaemia and hyperphosphataemia is typically seen with rhabdomyolysis. A grossly elevated troponin would indicate MI, but a lesser elevation would be non-specific. Similarly, a grossly elevated TSH level (>20 IU/L – normal range 0.4–5.0 mU/L) would indicate hypothyroidism, but a more modest increase would not be interpretable.

Urine

Dipstick for blood and protein. If positive for blood, check microscopy for red cells. A positive dipstick with no red cells is caused by urinary myoglobin in rhabdomyolysis.

Other tests

Chest radiograph; CT scan of the brain; blood (and other) cultures depending on clinical suspicion; and ABGs if patient very unwell.

Management

Any clear cause of bradycardia or complication of the collapse should be treated on its merits. But if the diagnosis is simply 'heart block' with no obvious precipitant that can be

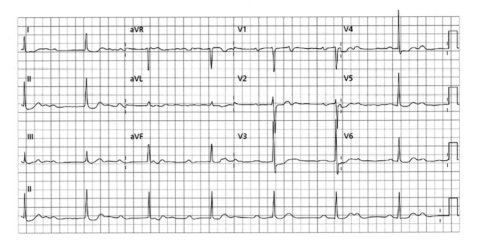

Fig 14 Complete heart block with a ventricular rate of 41 beats per minute: whether immediate pacing is required will depend on the clinical context.

removed, then management should depend on the state of the patient:

If the patient is well

Some patients can tolerate complete heart block at a pulse rate of 30 beats per minute if their left ventricular function is good. They may be fully conscious with a normal BP and warm peripheries. If this is the case, immediate transvenous pacing is not necessary and an elective decision on the need for a permanent pacing system can be taken. Close inpatient observation and cardiac monitoring is mandatory.

> **Key point**
>
> If a patient is tolerating their bradycardia, they almost certainly do not need temporary transvenous pacing.

If the patient is unwell

Immediate temporary cardiac pacing may be required if the patient is symptomatic. Marked bradyarrhythmia in someone who has suffered loss of consciousness – albeit transient – is almost certainly an indication for cardiac pacing; and the decision between a temporary transvenous procedure or the emergency insertion of

a permanent system will depend on local resources. Heart block with normal, narrow QRS complexes (<120 ms), as shown in Fig 14, suggests a nodal source of ventricular depolarisation and is less likely to require an immediate temporary pacemaker. Other treatments that may be helpful include:

> Atropine (initial dose of 0.5–1 mg IV) – this may speed up the patient's ventricular rate and buy time while temporary pacing is organised.

> Isoprenaline (infusion rate 2–10 μg/min IV, with a drug half-life of approximately 2 minutes) – may be useful *in extremis.*

> External cardiac pacemaker – may be used while arrangements are made for a definitive procedure, but patients will require sedation and analgesia.

Further comments

Bradycardia and myocardial infarction

The combination of AMI and bradyarrhythmia requiring temporary pacing presents a challenge, particularly as the bradycardia may resolve spontaneously with time. The procedure carries extra risk following thrombolysis, if used. Insert the pacing wire through the femoral vein so that pressure can be applied if there is bleeding, although this is impossible in the neck (the brachial is an alternative route, but manoeuvring the tip of the wire is often very difficult). If a wire has already been inserted through the internal jugular or subclavian vein in the context of AMI, most would then advocate that thrombolysis should not be undertaken.

Hypothermia

A core body temperature of less than 33°C is diagnostic of hypothermia (Fig 15). The management principles differ according to the cause of the lowered temperature:

> Rapid onset – in young patients the lowering of body temperature is often rapid, eg after immersion in water or collapse on a cold city street following alcohol intoxication: rapid ('active' or 'intensive') warming is required.

> Gradual onset – in most cases of hypothermia in older people the fall in body temperature occurs over several days, and so warming should be more gentle (warm bedding and a space blanket); indeed there is some evidence that intensive warming in older people causes cardiovascular collapse and arrhythmias.

Broad-spectrum antibiotics should be given empirically: pneumonia (both hypostatic and aspiration) is a complicating feature of abnormally low body temperature.

Hypothyroidism

Hypothyroidism is associated with a variety of bradyarrhythmias, particularly sinus bradycardia and AF with a slow ventricular rate. In acute, severe hypothyroidism steroids should be given before starting thyroid hormone replacement; without them, thyroid replacement therapy can result in acute circulatory collapse. Older patients often have coexisting ischaemic heart disease and their hypothyroidism will have developed over a considerable period of time. Vigorous replacement of thyroid hormone may well do more harm than

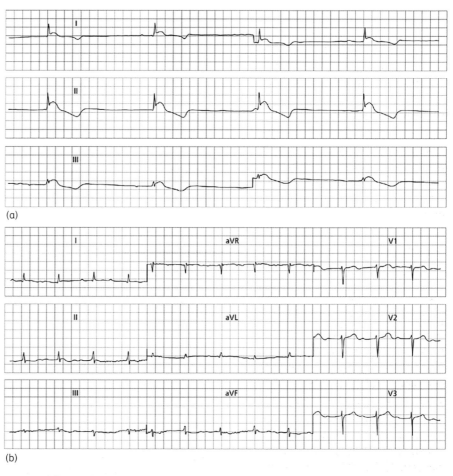

(a)

(b)

Fig 15 (a) ECG from a patient with a core temperature of 25°C, showing profound sinus bradycardia, first-degree heart block and prominent 'J'-waves; **(b)** ECG from the same patient after warming to 31°C, showing heart rate 75 beats per minute, persistent first-degree heart block and no 'J'-waves.

good, hence the starting dose of thyroxine should be very small, 25 µg daily, or even on alternate days. Triiodothyronine is rarely indicated.

Overdose with beta-blockers

Glucagon acts to reverse the effects of cardiovascular depression associated with beta-blocker overdose. The initial dosage is 5 mg, repeated as necessary. It may be necessary to start an infusion of glucagon if a long-acting beta-blocker has been taken – be aware that this necessitates dosing of glucagon that is very considerably higher than doses typically used in hypoglycaemia.

1.3.7 Asthma

Case history

A 36-year-old woman with a history of asthma since childhood is admitted with severe wheeze and breathlessness (respiratory rate 35 breaths per minute). You are asked to assess her in the emergency department resuscitation room. What treatment does she require? How will you decide if she needs input from the intensive care team?

Introduction

Undiagnosed, undertreated and poorly controlled asthma remain significant causes of mortality across the world. To prevent further deterioration, acute asthma attacks should always be promptly assessed, aggressively treated, and urgently escalated to intensive care (if required).

Key point

For all emergency cases – the history, examination and initial investigations should occur concurrently:

> Assess using the ABC approach.

> Start initial treatment – see below.

> Do you need to call for help immediately?

> If she looks dead or nearly dead – get help quickly.

> If she appears agitated or exhausted – get help quickly.

> Can she speak in full sentences, only in words or is she unable to speak? If only in words or unable to speak – get help quickly.

> Is she cyanosed or very hypoxic? If she is, she is nearly dead.

Assuming that your initial history, examination and investigations are consistent with the diagnosis of an acute exacerbation of asthma, then give oxygen, bronchodilators and steroids without delay:

> Oxygen – deliver inspired oxygen to maintain saturations of 94–98%.

> Bronchodilators – nebulised therapy should be given early and repeated frequently in the early stages of an acute attack: salbutamol 2.5–5.0 mg, repeated every 15–30 minutes until maximum 10 mg/h. This can be nebulised with anticholinergic drugs – ipratropium bromide (500 µg 4–6 hourly) – which gives additional benefit in acute asthma.

Hazard

Ensure that the nebuliser is driven by oxygen and not air!

> Steroids – give prednisolone 40–50 mg orally if the patient is able to take it. There is no evidence that intravenous hydrocortisone confers additional benefit in acute asthma, however if the patient is unable to swallow then give 200 mg stat followed by 400 mg daily (100 mg qds).

History of the presenting problem

The following questions are important in assessing the severity of and appropriate response to this attack:

> How long has she been breathless? There may be a short and fairly rapid deterioration; equally there may be a history of illness for a few days prior to admission in association with progressive breathlessness. Both sets of circumstances may be equally severe, but you would want to monitor much more closely the patient that seemed to be getting worse rapidly.

> Has she had variation in severity during the day or at night? Diurnal variation and nocturnal symptoms are important pointers to deterioration in asthmatics. Progressive and nocturnal symptoms probably indicate a loss of control of disease prior to presentation. If background control has been poor, recovery following treatment is often delayed.

> Has she been using more of her normal medication? If so, has it helped? Most asthmatics are familiar with their disease and will try and avoid coming to hospital. To avoid admission, they often self-medicate with increasing amounts until a point at which it no longer helps.

> Although the presumption is that the problem is due to an attack of asthma, are there any features that are unusual? Has she been feverish to suggest a precipitating infection? Has she had pleuritic chest pain that may indicate a spontaneous pneumothorax? Is she pregnant, and is this actually a pulmonary embolus?

> Are you able to identify any precipitant for her asthma attack? Has she got new carpets or pets at home? Has she not been using her medication? Has she recently come off steroids?

Other relevant history

It will be important to establish how well/poorly controlled her asthma usually is, and whether or not she monitors it:

> How debilitating is her asthma normally, and what can't she do because of it? Does she ever measure her peak flow, and if so, what are her usual readings?

> How frequently does she have attacks of asthma, and how bad have they been? How many times has she needed to see her GP or to be admitted to hospital in the last 12 months? When was her last course of steroids? Has she ever needed to be admitted to a high-dependency unit (HDU) or to an ICU, and has she ever needed artificial ventilation? These are always worrying features.

> What medication does she take normally? The need for home nebulisers and/or maintenance steroids probably signifies poorly controlled or 'brittle asthma'. In addition to any medication she may be taking for her asthma, it is important to ask whether she is on any other new medications, or if she has recently received antibiotics or steroids in the community.

Examination

The British Thoracic Society / Scottish Intercollegiate Guidelines Network (BTS/SIGN) guidelines for assessing the severity of acute asthma are given in Table 6.

Respiratory

Respiratory rate – it is important to measure respiratory rate, but the degree of tachypnoea does not correlate with the severity of an asthma attack. Asthma is a terrifying condition and most acute asthmatics hyperventilate, but then their respiratory rate falls as they become exhausted with the effort of breathing – eventually leading to hypercapnic respiratory failure and the need for ventilatory support.

Hazard
Respiratory rate must be interpreted in the context of the whole patient – a normal respiratory rate is consistent with imminent death in the asthmatic who is becoming exhausted.

Widespread wheezing indicates airways obstruction, but beware the asthmatic who has a silent chest on auscultation – the tidal volume may be reduced so much that insufficient flow is being generated to create a wheeze. Check for signs of an underlying pneumothorax and for pneumonic consolidation.

Cardiovascular

Sinus tachycardia is common in acute asthma and does not correlate with severity. Fear, increased sympathetic drive and bronchodilator drugs all contribute to a rise in pulse rate. Bradycardia may supervene as hypoxia becomes more marked.

The degree of pulsus paradoxus (which is an exaggeration of the normal fall in systolic BP on inspiration) does correlate with severity of asthma as it reflects the abnormal changes in transpulmonary pressure generated by increasing airways obstruction.

Hazard
No clinical sign correlates well with the degree of hypoxia – measure ABGs at the earliest opportunity!

Investigations

> Peak flow – Is she too tired/breathless to attempt this? How does the value now compare to her usual one, and how do you interpret the result (see Table 6)?

> Pulse oximetry – will be useful in detection of hypoxia, but the absence of hypoxia does not guarantee that all is well.

Hazard
Oximetry only gives part of the picture – it quantifies arterial oxygenation but does not tell you how well a patient is ventilating. A patient given high-flow oxygen might not be hypoxic but could still be hypoventilating and be at risk of respiratory arrest.

> ABGs – mandatory in all cases of life-threatening asthma or where the saturations are <92%. Initially you may see slight hypoxia/normoxia with reduced $PaCO_2$, suggesting hyperventilation in order to maintain adequate oxygenation. Hypoxia, hypercapnia and acidosis ensue as the patient tires. A metabolic acidosis in acute asthma is a bad prognostic sign, suggesting impaired cardiac output due to severe airflow obstruction.

Table 6	The BTS / SIGN guidelines (2016) for assessing the severity of acute asthma
Severity	**Features**
Acute severe asthma	PEFR 33–50% of best (use % predicted if best unknown) Cannot complete sentences in one breath Respiratory rate >25 breaths per minute Pulse >110 beats per minute
Life threatening	PEFR <33% of best or predicted SpO_2 <92% or PaO_2 <8 kPa Normal $PaCO_2$ 4.6–6.0 kPa Silent chest, cyanosis or feeble respiratory effort Bradycardia, arrhythmia or hypotension Exhaustion, confusion or coma
Near fatal asthma	Raised $PaCO_2$ Requiring intermittent positive-pressure ventilation with raised inflation pressures

BTS, British Thoracic Society; $PaCO_2$, partial pressure of carbon dioxide in arterial blood; PaO_2, partial pressure of oxygen in arterial blood; PEFR, peak expiratory flow rate; SIGN, Scottish Intercollegiate Guidelines Network; SpO_2, peripheral capillary oxygen saturation.

Key point

Most patients with asthma hate having ABGs taken due to previous bad experiences. A 22G needle is perfectly adequate, rather than a 20G or even an 18G. If local anaesthetic is required, warm it up to reduce the stinging.

> Chest radiograph – this is not required in every case but should be arranged unless you are confident the patient does not have a pneumothorax, consolidation due to superadded infection or segmental collapse due to sputum plugging.
> Routine blood investigations – FBC (anaemia will compound impaired tissue oxygen delivery) and electrolytes (β_2-agonists, theophyllines and steroids all predispose to hypokalaemia, which can create a respiratory myopathy).
> ECG – sinus tachycardia will be the likely finding, but it is important to exclude any tachyarrhythmias that may result primarily as a result of cardiac compromise or secondarily to treatment strategies (ie β_2-agonists or theophyllines).

Management

What do you do if the patient does not improve?

Key point

It is vital that senior clinician support and ICU support is requested sooner rather than later – do not delay: asthmatics can deteriorate rapidly.

So far the patient has been treated with oxygen, bronchodilators and steroids. However, if life-threatening features are present, or the patient does not improve after 15–30 minutes, then further treatments need to be administered with senior supervision:

> Intravenous magnesium sulphate – 1.2–2.0 g over 20 minutes. This works as a calcium antagonist that induces smooth muscle relaxation. Studies show a somewhat mixed response, but a single dose of intravenous magnesium sulphate has been shown to be effective and safe in acute severe asthma by improving lung function and reducing intubation rates. Do not give repeated doses.
> Intravenous bronchodilators – aminophylline should be used with caution, especially if oral theophyllines are part of the patient's regular medication. The potential complications of aminophylline toxicity – arrhythmias, epileptic convulsions and/or vomiting – are extremely dangerous in acute asthma (5 mg/kg loading dose over 20 minutes, then infusion of 0.5–0.7 mg/kg/h to keep plasma level 10–20 mg/L). Salbutamol is an alternative – dilute 5 mg in 500 mL, 5% dextrose or 0.9% saline, and start infusion at a rate of 7.5 µg/min, titrating according to response. The main side effects are tachycardia and tremor.

Hazard

β_2-agonists and aminophylline must always be given with oxygen, not instead of it. These drugs are pulmonary vasodilators as well as bronchodilators and their administration can rapidly worsen the ventilation/perfusion mismatch, causing a reduction in arterial oxygen tension unless supplemental oxygen is given.

> Intravenous fluids – hyperventilation and poor oral intake can lead to dehydration. Dry bronchial secretions are more difficult to clear and can lead to sputum plugging. A relatively high right ventricular filling pressure is necessary in patients with severe airways obstruction to safeguard cardiac output. Do not be frightened to give 1 L crystalloid in the first 1–2 hours. Also be aware that repeated doses of salbutamol can cause hypokalaemia and therefore electrolyte replacement is required.
> Antibiotics are not routinely indicated unless there is good evidence of a bacterial infection. Most infections which precede asthma attacks are viral in nature.

Regular clinical reassessment of the patient is crucial, supplemented by repeated measurement of peak expiratory flow rate (PEFR) 15–30 minutes after commencing treatment, oximetry and ABG measurements.

Further comments

Patients with asthma still die. It is important to remember that early review by the ICU is important. If the patient is admitted *in extremis* or does not improve with treatment, get help. The move to the ICU should be a cool elective decision, not a panic when the patient is close to a respiratory arrest. Important pointers to a deterioration may include:

> if a patient has required previous admission to an ICU/HDU
> exhaustion, feeble respirations, confusion or drowsiness
> deteriorating PEFR
> worsening or persisting hypoxia or hypercapnia.

1.3.8 Pleurisy

Case history

A 22-year-old woman is referred to the emergency department because of the sudden onset of a right-sided, pleuritic chest pain. She has no previous medical or surgical history. She has taken the oral contraceptive pill for the past 12 months. Her GP writes 'I would be grateful if you could exclude a pulmonary embolus as the cause of her symptoms'.

Introduction

This is a pulmonary embolus until proved otherwise.

Priorities are:

> Airway, breathing and circulation (ABC).

> Is the patient ill? If so, administer high-flow oxygen and monitor pulse oximetry; check her respiratory rate, heart rate and BP; obtain intravenous access; and give fluid bolus if the patient is hypotensive. Cardiovascular collapse indicates massive PE and is an indication for thrombolysis – call for senior help earlier rather than later.

> Low-molecular-weight heparin – this should be administered without delay to protect against further embolisation in all patients with a high probability of PE. Doctors often delay giving heparin until they have completed taking the history, examined the patient and obtained the result of initial investigations.

> Analgesia – pleurisy is painful! Relieve the pain as soon as possible. NSAIDs are excellent for relieving the pain of pleurisy, but opiates may be required as well.

Key point

If it is clear that PE is the number one diagnosis – start treatment immediately unless there are obvious pressing contraindications.

History of presenting problem

Look specifically for features in the history that would point to a diagnosis of PE:

> Pain – did it start suddenly or gradually? The former is typical of PE, but a gradual onset of symptoms does not exclude the diagnosis. Sudden onset of pain (and/or breathlessness) after defaecation is highly suggestive of PE, and there is commonly a story of becoming suddenly very frightened (a sense of impending doom).

> Breathlessness – autopsy studies show that patients who die of PE virtually always have evidence that PEs have occurred over a period of time: has she had recent breathlessness or had to slow down?

> Haemoptysis – the commonest differential diagnosis of pleurisy is musculoskeletal pain, and this does not cause haemoptysis.

> Calf/leg swelling or pain – these would suggest DVT and strongly support the diagnosis of PE in this clinical context.

> Has the patient had a DVT or PE before?

> Is there a major risk factor? Ask about recent immobility/major surgery/lower limb trauma or surgery, pregnancy/post-partum, any major medical illness, taking oral contraceptives (as in this case) and a family history of such illnesses.

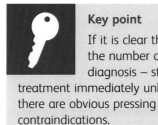

Hazard

Pitfall in the diagnosis of pulmonary embolism (PE)

Pleuritic pain is not always a feature of PE – large, central emboli typically cause cardiovascular collapse and breathlessness; smaller, more peripheral emboli tend to cause pain.

Key point

Differential diagnosis of pleurisy:

> Spontaneous pneumothorax – heparin can convert this into a haemothorax!

> Pneumonia – fever is often a prominent symptom, and chest signs and radiography will usually show consolidation. However, fever and radiographic consolidation can be a feature of pulmonary infarction.

> Musculoskeletal pain – this can be difficult to differentiate. If the diagnosis is unclear, anticoagulate until PE is excluded.

> Less common and rare conditions – pain indistinguishable from pleurisy can be due to shingles (herpes zoster), and pleurisy can be the presenting symptom of systemic lupus erythematosus (check the relevant serology – antinuclear factor and DNA binding – and be particularly suspicious if pleurisy is recurrent).

Also remember that the presenting history (and findings) in PE may be dominated by secondary cardiac features – ischaemic cardiac pain and ECG changes. A PE creates a sudden increase in afterload on the right ventricle, and 'secondary cardiac pain' from the resulting myocardial ischaemia may be a prominent feature of the history.

Examination

The first priority will clearly be to make an assessment of the severity of illness (as described in Section 1.3.2); but with regard to the particular diagnosis of PE, proceed as follows.

Cardiovascular

Heart rate – the most common sign is sinus tachycardia; BP – may be elevated due to catecholamine release or may be reduced secondary to cardiovascular collapse; but most importantly look for signs of pulmonary hypertension:

> Elevated venous pressure, particularly with an exaggerated 'a'-wave.

> Right ventricular heave – which can develop surprisingly rapidly following an acute rise in pulmonary artery pressure.

> Right ventricular gallop rhythm and loud pulmonary second sound.

Respiratory

Most patients with a PE have respiratory rate >20 breaths per minute; but more specifically:

> Added sounds – a pleural rub may be present. Always believe other medical staff if they describe a rub that is no longer present when you examine the patient.

Hazard

Chest wall tenderness

Patients with PE will tell you that it has been uncomfortable lying on the affected side and they may be locally tender on palpation. This is an important point because local tenderness does not necessarily mean pain of musculoskeletal origin – another classic diagnostic 'catch'.

Other features

Search for a DVT, but do not be surprised if you do not find one. Also, do not let its absence put you off making the diagnosis of PE. A rectal examination (and pelvic and breast examination in women) will be necessary at some stage, but not on admission of a patient who is breathless and unwell.

Investigation

Routine tests

All patients with this history require:

> Chest radiograph – in PE the findings are usually normal, but a number of radiographic abnormalities may occur: line shadows at the bases; peripheral wedge-shaped shadow(s); areas of relative oligaemia in the lung fields (rare); and enlarged proximal pulmonary artery (rare).

> ECG – in PE the ECG is commonly normal but it may show: sinus tachycardia; T-wave inversion in V1–V3; an 'S1Q3T3' pattern – commonly described in medical literature and reflecting axis change as a result of a sudden increase in right ventricular afterload (Fig 16); right atrial hypertrophy with a 'P pulmonale'; right bundle branch block (can be a normal variant, but is significant if new); and evidence of ischaemic change – which may be left- or right-sided.

Other tests that may be appropriate include:

> D-dimer – only a negative result is of any value, hence It should only be measured where there is reasonable clinical suspicion of PE, but not where an alternative diagnosis is highly likely (when a 'positive' D-dimer will almost inevitably be a false positive) or if the clinical probability of a PE is high (when the patient requires a definitive investigation, whatever the D-dimer result might be). In this case it would only be appropriate for you to measure a D-dimer if you thought 'if this test is negative, I will reassure the woman, treat her symptomatically, and send her home'.

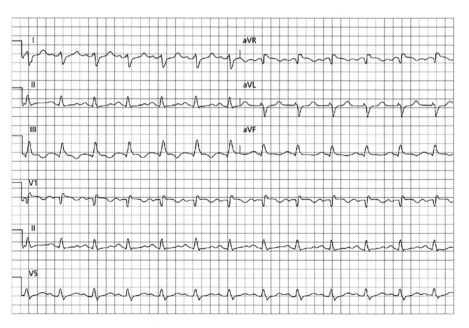

Fig 16 An ECG in a case of acute PE showing the 'S1Q3T3' pattern.

Key point

D-dimer is very helpful if used wisely – but it should not be used as a routine screening test for PE in patients with a low probability of the condition. Doing so will inevitably generate a large number of false-positive results.

> Blood gases – these typically show hypocapnia in PE because of hyperventilation. Hypoxia may or may not be present. If there is a base deficit, your concerns should be heightened because it indicates secondary cardiovascular compromise. Calculation of the alveolar–arterial gradient may be helpful.

Definitive investigations

Computed tomography (CT) pulmonary angiography is now the imaging modality of choice (Fig 17).

Ventilation/perfusion isotope lung scan may be considered as the initial imaging investigation provided the chest radiograph is normal, there is no significant cardiopulmonary disease,

standardised reporting criteria are used and a non-diagnostic result is always followed by further imaging. The presence of chronic lung or cardiac disease makes interpretation of ventilation/perfusion scans very difficult if not impossible (Fig 18).

Other tests

Routine haematological and biochemical tests should be performed: are there any clues to a systemic disease that might predispose to PE? A leg ultrasound scan is an alternative definitive imaging modality where there is a clinical

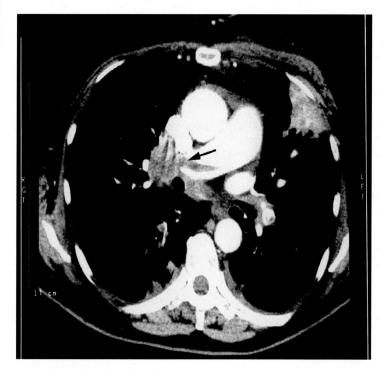

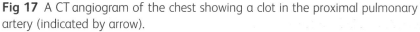

Fig 17 A CT angiogram of the chest showing a clot in the proximal pulmonary artery (indicated by arrow).

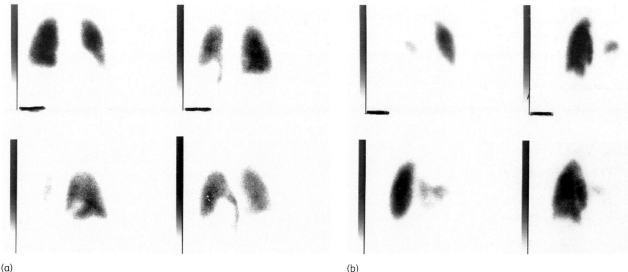

(a)   (b)

Fig 18 Pulmonary emboli (PE) revealed on perfusion isotope lung scanning: **(a)** large, segmental defect in the left lung; **(b)** virtually complete lack of perfusion in the right lung. Ventilation scanning was normal in both patients.

suspicion of a DVT, because identification of a DVT precludes the need for further tests. A patient with a proven DVT and pleuritic pain should be treated as if they have a PE (because it is virtually impossible to think that they have not had one). There is a role for echocardiography in an unstable patient in whom the clinical suspicion of PE is high.

Hazard
It is not possible to interpret the results of a thrombophilia screen in the presence of thrombus or anticoagulation.

Management

Anticoagulation/thrombolysis
Low-molecular-weight heparin followed by warfarin will be appropriate for most patients, although in some situations long-term low-molecular-weight heparin is more appropriate eg in those with active cancer. Direct oral anticoagulants (DOACs), such as rivaroxaban, are increasingly being used in place of warfarin.

In some cases, thrombolytic agents will be indicated. There is no trial evidence to guide decision making, but a common view would be that thrombolysis is indicated in patients with circulatory collapse, or those who are persistently hypotensive from embolic disease despite initial anticoagulation. Alteplase is typically given as a 10 mg bolus, followed by an infusion of 50–90 mg over 2 hours (dependent on body weight) in those with circulatory collapse, or a bolus of 50 mg (repeated if necessary) in those with cardiac arrest due to PE – but do follow local guidelines if there are any.

Other aspects
If there is significant haemodynamic disturbance, then a high venous filling pressure is required to assist the struggling right ventricle. Give intravenous fluid (500 mL) swiftly and reassess. Close haemodynamic monitoring is required, ideally in a HDU or ICU, so that deterioration can be spotted promptly and thrombolysis administered.

Repeated embolic events despite adequate anticoagulation may require mechanical intervention, eg insertion of a filter device into the inferior vena cava.

In patients with no clear risk factors consider investigations for underlying conditions: PE may also be the first presentation of a malignancy.

Key point
Take home messages regarding PEs are:

> They are a common and potentially life-threatening condition.

> The presentation is often atypical – if confronted with unexplained breathlessness or collapse, always consider the possibility of PE.

> Do not expect to find a predisposing cause for venous thrombosis.

> Examination is commonly unremarkable.

> The chest radiograph and ECG are commonly normal.

> CT angiography and ventilation/ perfusion scans are particularly valuable soon after the clinical event – normal images obtained more than 48 hours after the clinical event do not exclude PE.

> Anticoagulate promptly while investigations are organised and the diagnosis is clarified. Give heparin. If the patient is very ill, do not hesitate to seek senior advice – the next PE may be fatal – and consider thrombolysis.

1.3.9 Chest infection/pneumonia

Case history
A 68-year-old woman with no significant past medical history is sent to the medical assessment unit with a 48-hour history of fever, malaise, breathlessness and progressive confusion. The note from the referring GP suggests that she thinks the problem is pneumonia. You are asked to assess her.

History of the presenting problem
Pneumonia does seem the most likely diagnosis in this case; hence pursue the symptoms described above and others that might be found in this condition:

> Fever – a low-grade fever is non-specific, but a fever of over 38.5°C in this context clearly supports pneumonia or another infective cause of illness (see Sections 1.3.25 and 1.3.30), as would the presence of rigors or 'chills'.

> Breathlessness – clearly supports the diagnosis of pneumonia, suggesting that there has been some ventilation–perfusion mismatch as may be seen with pneumonic consolidation.

> Cough – is there a cough, and is it productive, purulent or dry? And does the woman normally have a cough and/or produce sputum? In the patient with normal lungs a dry cough is a common presenting feature of pneumonia of any sort; a purulent cough is indicative of an underlying bacterial infection; and brownish-red (rusty coloured) sputum most likely due to pneumococcal infection.

> Chest pain – this may simply be due to 'sore ribs' from coughing or it may be pleuritic, which is more common in bacterial than non-bacterial infection.

> When did the illness start? The information given here suggests it was in the past 48 hours, but it is important to try and pinpoint the onset of symptoms or the prodromal stage of the illness. Non-bacterial causes of pneumonia (ie *Mycoplasma pneumoniae*) are often characterised by a relatively long prodromal stage in comparison to bacterial pneumonias.

> Confusion – indicates that the pneumonia is likely to be severe (see below), but note that the classic symptoms and signs of pneumonia are less likely in older patients and so confusion may be the main presenting feature and only diagnostic clue.

> Is any other diagnosis more likely? Other common causes of acute presentation with breathlessness are pulmonary oedema or pulmonary embolism (PE): are there features to support either of these diagnoses? See Sections 1.3.2 and 1.3.8 for discussion. Remember that patients with atypical pneumonia commonly have gastrointestinal symptoms.

Other relevant history

A detailed past medical history is required, but issues of particular relevance are:

> Previous respiratory disease – does she have known chronic obstructive pulmonary disease (COPD), bronchiectasis or any other long-standing lung problems?

> Smoking history.

> Alcohol history – alcoholism may predispose the patient to aspiration as well as pneumococcal, Gram-negative and atypical infections. In addition, it is important to recognise if a patient is likely to suffer from alcohol withdrawal if admitted to hospital.

> Pets – is there a parrot or budgie at home?

> Is she immunosuppressed or has she had a splenectomy?

> Always consider the possibility of HIV, particularly in younger patients without other risk factors for pneumonia.

Examination

A woman with pneumonia sufficient to cause delirium is likely to be very ill. Proceed as indicated in Section 1.3.2, but noting especially in the chest – are there signs of consolidation? A pleural rub, crepitations, bronchial breathing or reduced breath sounds from a parapneumonic effusion are all suggestive of bacterial pneumonia.

Hazard

Remember that in non-bacterial pneumonia the respiratory signs are commonly unimpressive.

Investigation

Pulse oximetry/arterial blood gases

Oximetry is mandatory in all patients: those with SaO_2 <92% or features of severe pneumonia should have arterial blood gas (ABG) measurements. A rising

$PaCO_2$ indicates failing ventilation – often as a consequence of patient exhaustion – and is a very worrying sign that should immediately trigger a request for senior support/ICU input or both.

Hazard

Measurement of oxygen saturation by pulse oximetry is likely to be inaccurate if there is poor peripheral perfusion – an instance when the early assessment of ABG is essential. Always document the inspired oxygen content when the ABG was taken.

Chest radiograph

Pneumococcal pneumonia presents classically as lobar or segmental consolidation (Fig 19). Multiple, non-contiguous and sometimes bilateral segments may be affected, with multilobar involvement being a poor prognostic factor. The absence of an 'air bronchogram' within an area of consolidation suggests exudate or pus filling the conducting airways; aside from *Streptococcus pneumoniae*, organisms commonly responsible for this

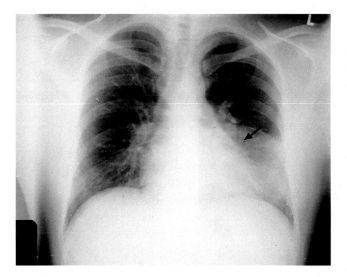

Fig 19 Lingular consolidation due to pneumococcus: the arrow marks an air bronchogram.

appearance are *Staphylococcus* (Fig 20) and Gram negatives. Early cavitation in an area of consolidation is typical of staphylococcal infection, but consider Gram negatives such as *Klebsiella* and do not forget *Mycobacterium tuberculosis* – although this does not cause acute illness. Also consider aspiration pneumonia or proximal bronchial obstruction, eg due to carcinoma or a foreign body. A variety of radiographic patterns are described in *Mycoplasma* pneumonia (Fig 21) and in Legionnaires' disease. The presence of pleural fluid is suggestive of bacterial aetiology and a diagnostic tap should be performed if this is anything more than trivial in size.

Hazard

In *Streptococcus pneumoniae* pneumonia the radiograph may be normal at presentation – even in the presence of a classical history and signs of consolidation on examination – only to become abnormal over the next few hours.

Routine blood tests

Full blood count

Anaemia will compound impaired tissue oxygen delivery and the white cell count is likely to be elevated. However, a patient with overwhelming sepsis may have a normal white cell count.

Electrolytes and renal function tests

Uraemia is a bad prognostic sign in pneumonia (see below, CURB-65); hyponatraemia is another non-specific marker of the severity of illness, but is also (for unknown reasons) a particular feature of Legionnaires' disease.

Liver blood tests

Derangement of liver enzymes may be seen in any severe sepsis, but note that

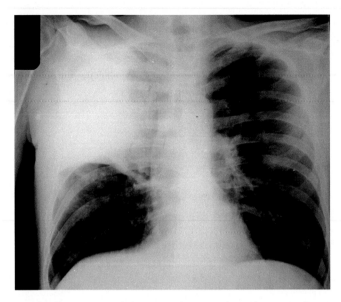

Fig 20 Dense consolidation with no air bronchogram due to staphylococcal pneumonia following flu.

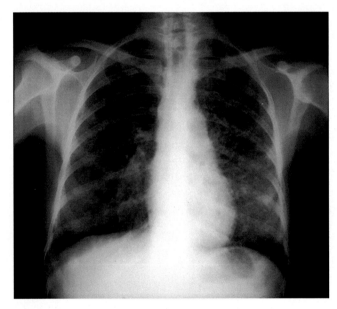

Fig 21 *Mycoplasma* pneumonia showing a lobular pattern of consolidation.

transient hepatitis is seen as part of multisystem involvement in atypical infections (ie Legionnaires' disease). Also pay attention to inflammatory markers, ie C-reactive protein (CRP) – a raised CRP on admission is a relatively more sensitive marker of pneumonia than an increased temperature or raised white cell count.

Microbiological tests

These include:

> sputum microscopy and culture – if sputum is obtainable it is important to send a sample early in the illness; also do this for acid-fast bacilli if clinically indicated

> blood cultures

> urinary assays of specific antigens – pneumococcal antigen and *Legionella* antigen

> serological testing – send acute and convalescent titres for atypical serology

> pleural fluid, if there is significant effusion.

Management

General management and resuscitation (if required) should be as described in Section 1.3.2, but note the following.

Key point

The CURB-65 Score (BTS guideline 2009) assessment is vital as a prognostic indicator:

> confusion – Mini Mental State Examination <8, or new disorientation in person, place and time

> urea – >7 mmol/L

> respiratory rate – >30 breaths per minute

> BP – systolic BP <90 mmHg or diastolic BP <60 mmHg

> age >65 years.

Score 1 point for each feature present; 3–5 suggests severe pneumonia.

Antibiotics

Antibiotics should be given without delay, with the choice guided by the BTS Guidelines and/or local knowledge of resistance patterns of the pathogens that are most commonly implicated. By a considerable margin, *Streptococcus*

pneumoniae is the commonest pathogen in community-acquired pneumonia. Always consult local prescribing policies in addition to obtaining microbiological advice as necessary.

> A CURB-65 score 1 or 2 – in the moderately sick patient, oral amoxicillin and a macrolide should be given. In those patients allergic to penicillin, a fluoroquinolone should be considered (ie levofloxacin).

> A CURB-65 score 3 or more – in the more severely ill patient, co-amoxiclav or a third-generation cephalosporin should be given intravenously in conjunction with a macrolide. In patients who are penicillin allergic, an intravenous fluoroquinolone in addition to a macrolide should be considered.

> If Legionnaires' disease is suspected, then intravenous erythromycin 1 g 6-hourly should be included.

> If there is the suggestion of preceding influenza, consider adding a specific antistaphylococcal antibiotic, eg flucloxacillin.

> If Gram-negative infection or aspiration is suspected, then a third-generation cephalosporin is the antibiotic of choice.

Further comments

Remember that patients with severe pneumonia have high insensible losses due to hyperventilation and fever in addition to reduced oral intake: they may require up to 4 L/day of intravenous fluid, with careful clinical examination at least twice daily to ensure that they are not becoming volume deplete or overloaded. This approach needs to be balanced against the particular requirements

of older patients who may have cardiovascular disease and heart failure, necessitating a more cautious fluid replacement strategy.

Radiograph changes are not static and the radiograph may deteriorate during the early stages of treatment. However, if the radiograph deteriorates despite antibiotic therapy, you may not be covering the correct organism or the diagnosis of infection may be incorrect. Consider other pathologies, such as pulmonary infarction, pulmonary eosinophilia, cryptogenic organising pneumonia or pulmonary vasculitis.

1.3.10 Acute on chronic airways obstruction

Case history

A 68-year-old man with a 50-pack-year history of smoking and known COPD has had increasing cough and breathlessness for the last 7 days and now presents to the emergency department. You are asked to assess him.

History of the presenting problem

You need to establish his normal level of respiratory function and the cause and severity of this deterioration.

Normal level of respiratory function and severity of deterioration

What is his usual exercise tolerance? How far can he normally walk? Can he climb a flight of stairs without stopping? How has his exercise capacity changed now? See the Medical Research Council dyspnoea scale below.

Grade of breathlessness related to activities:

1 Not troubled by breathlessness, except on strenuous exercise.

2 Short of breath when hurrying or walking up a slight hill.

3 Walks slower than most people on the level, stops after a mile, or stops after 15 minutes walking at own pace.

4 Stops for breath after walking about 100 metres, or after a few minutes on level ground.

5 Too breathless to leave the house, or breathless when dressing or undressing.

Cause of deterioration

The most likely explanation for deterioration is an acute exacerbation of COPD, but do not neglect to consider other possibilities. Important aspects of history to pursue are:

> What is his normal treatment, and has this been increased recently? How many exacerbations does he have each year? Ask particularly about steroids, recent courses of antibiotics, home nebulisers and home oxygen/ventilation.

> Fever / increase in sputum production / change in sputum colour suggest an infective process.

> Chest pain – pleuritic pain could be due to pneumonia or fracture of a rib through coughing.

Also consider whether there could there be another diagnosis: heavy smokers are clearly at risk of coronary heart disease and thereby left ventricular failure. How many pillows does the patient normally sleep with? Does he normally wake up at night due to breathlessness? Is this different from normal now? Do not overinterpret orthopnoea and paroxysmal nocturnal dyspnoea because any patient with respiratory difficulty will find it more difficult to breathe when lying down, but remember that left ventricular failure and COPD commonly coexist. Are there any features to suggest PE (see Section 1.3.8)? Could he have a pneumothorax (see Section 1.3.12)?

Other relevant history

A thorough past medical history is required, and also careful scrutiny of the patient's hospital notes (if available), with issues of particular relevance being:

> The number of admissions with respiratory problems in the past 5 years.

> What treatments were required on those admissions (specifically has he ever needed non-invasive ventilation (NIV) or invasive ventilation)?

> Social circumstances, including suitability of accommodation, will be important in considering discharge planning. Would this patient be suitable for the 'hospital at home / supported discharge' service available in many hospitals for patients with exacerbations of COPD?

Examination

As always, this should begin with an assessment of the overall severity of illness, as described in Section 1.3.2, with particular emphasis on two questions: 'What is the degree of respiratory distress?', and 'Can

pneumothorax be excluded?' Hence look in particular for the following:

> Can the patient speak in sentences or just a few words at a time?

> Do they look exhausted?

> Are they using accessory muscles?

> Are they cyanosed?

> What is their respiratory rate? However, remember that a 'normal' respiratory rate is not a reassuring finding in a patient that is becoming exhausted. An examination of the chest is likely to reveal scattered wheezes and crackles, but beware the silent chest and note if there is any consolidation suggesting pneumonia. Look in the sputum pot and check the PEFR.

Investigations

As in Section 1.3.9, but pay particular attention to the following:

> Arterial blood gas (ABG) – prompt assessment is particularly important in this case because of the possibility that this patient might have type 2 respiratory failure with a high PCO_2. A high PCO_2 with a normal pH suggests chronic ventilatory failure, with an elevated bicarbonate level due to renal compensation.

> Chest radiograph – look specifically for a pneumothorax and/or focal lung pathology, which may be the result of infective consolidation or a bronchial carcinoma.

> Blood tests – as well as those detailed in Section 1.3.9, check the theophylline level in patients on theophylline at admission.

> If sputum is purulent this should be sent for microscopy and culture.

Management

If the patient is *in extremis*, then resuscitation should proceed as described in Section 1.3.2.

Key point

If a patient with known COPD looks very ill or worse, they should be given high-flow oxygen to buy time for rapid assessment and instigation of ventilatory support – as stated before: hypoxia kills, hypercarbia merely intoxicates.

Management in a less severe case comprises:

> Oxygen – in patients who are not about to die, controlled O_2 (starting with 24%, given via a humidifier) is administered according to the ABG findings, aiming to get the SaO_2 >92%. The ABG should be rechecked within 60 minutes of starting O_2 therapy and again within 60 minutes of a change in inspired O_2. Humidification is important to decrease mucous plugging.

> Bronchodilators – nebulised β_2-agonist (eg salbutamol 5 mg) and anticholinergic (eg ipratropium 500 mcg), repeated as necessary. Remember that the driving gas for nebulised therapy should be specified. In hypercapnia the

nebuliser should be driven by air rather than oxygen.

> Steroids – start oral steroids (eg prednisolone 30 mg for 7 days). Consider whether a tapering dose of steroids is required. If patients are unable to take oral steroids then IV hydrocortisone can be used.

> Antibiotics should be given if there is a history of more purulent sputum / consolidation on chest X-ray / clinical evidence of pneumonia. (Choice of antibiotic according to local guidelines.)

> Chest physiotherapy – to help with sputum expectoration; but will not be helpful if the patient has a very tight chest and is not coughing anything up.

Key point

Patients with asthma or COPD produce thick viscous secretions that significantly contribute to airway obstruction and are difficult to clear. Humidification of air/oxygen is simple, has no adverse side effects, and helps greatly – so do not forget it.

Non-invasive ventilation

Non-invasive ventilation (NIV) has been shown to reduce mortality in COPD patients presenting with decompensated respiratory acidosis. BTS guidelines recommend:

> NIV should be considered in any patient in whom respiratory acidosis (pH <7.35) persists despite medical treatment after a maximum of 1 hour (controlled oxygen, salbutamol and ipratropium).

> Patients who are more unwell (eg pH <7.26) should be managed in a HDU or ICU with a low threshold for intubation if appropriate.

> An ABG should be repeated 1 hour after initiation of NIV and after any change in settings.

> A management plan in the event of deterioration should be made at the time NIV is commenced and ceiling of therapy should be documented.

> In patients not improving on NIV within 4 hours, intubation and mechanical ventilation should be considered if appropriate.

If confronted with a moribund patient in whom a decision has not already been made, then the default position must clearly be to proceed with treatment. However, efforts should be made to discuss management with a respiratory physician if possible, preferably one who already knows the patient.

(Further details on NIV are described in Section 3.8).

1.3.11 Stridor

Case history

A 64-year-old woman who is a lifelong heavy smoker is brought to the emergency department with a history of progressive shortness of breath and 'noisy breathing'. She has been unwell for a couple of months, complains of generalised lethargy and weakness, and has lost weight. You are asked to see her urgently as the triage nurse thinks she has stridor.

Introduction

Key point

Priorities in the management of someone with suspected stridor are:

> Check ABC (airway, breathing and circulation).

> Get help early – you need someone with anaesthetic skills and possibly ears, nose and throat expertise.

> Give 100% oxygen and obtain intravenous access.

> Do NOT attempt to look at the patient's airway in any greater detail than by carefully looking in the front of the mouth for any obvious blockage (eg dental plate); do NOT ask the patient to open their mouth as wide as possible; and do NOT put your fingers in 'hunting for something'.

> Let the patient determine their best position – often patients are sitting up, trying to manage their own airway. Getting them to lie flat may quickly change a borderline airway to a blocked one.

> Consider the presumptive diagnosis (Table 7) and start treatment based on this.

History of the presenting problem

The patient may not be able to speak, in which case the history may be available from someone else, but important features to consider are as follows.

Speed of onset

Aspiration of a foreign body may present suddenly with a history of coughing or choking; in acute anaphylaxis stridor is of sudden onset and can be quickly progressive; hoarseness and shortness of breath with systemic deterioration of more insidious onset (as in this case) is more

Table 7	Causes of stridor	
Cause	**Common example**	**Less common or rare example**
Intrinsic narrowing of airway	Aspiration of a foreign body	Acute pharyngitis / laryngitis / retropharyngeal abscess
	Anaphylaxis	Laryngeal trauma
	Epiglottitis (especially in children)	Inhalation injury
	Laryngeal tumour	
Extrinsic compression of airway	Mediastinal tumour	Mediastinal lymphadenopathy
	Retrosternal thyroid	

suggestive of an underlying tumour; and patients with a retrosternal thyroid enlargement may present with slow onset of dysphagia and hoarseness that predate the presentation of stridor.

Exacerbating or triggering factors

Although not likely in this case with a history that seems to be of 2 months' duration, is there a history of a bee sting or other allergen exposure that may result in anaphylaxis? Is there a history of smoke inhalation, which may cause laryngeal oedema and bronchospasm within 48 hours of exposure? Was there a history of a prodromal viral/infective illness or sore throat that could suggest acute laryngitis or epiglottitis? Is there a history of intubation, bronchoscopy or laryngoscopy, all of which may result in laryngeal trauma, oedema or spasm? Is there a history of previous neck surgery or tracheostomy?

Other relevant history

Is there a history of known malignancy? This may be the first presentation of this patient with this malignancy, but it is important to find out if there is a history of thoracic or laryngeal malignancy, either of which may have progressed. Does the patient have a condition that could cause recurrent aspiration, eg motor neurone disease or progressive supranuclear palsy?

Examination

Key point

If the patient is *in extremis*, put out a cardiac arrest call immediately.

If the patient has stridor but is clinically stable and does not seem to be in danger of imminent catastrophe, then look for the following:

> Clubbing – would strongly suggest a malignant cause in this clinical context.

> Lymphadenopathy – enlarged cervical lymph nodes may be present in malignancy.

> Evidence of trauma – bruising or palpable subcutaneous crepitus in the neck.

> Signs of thyrotoxicosis, thyroid enlargement or the presence of a retrosternal thyroid.

> Distended and non-pulsatile neck veins – suggesting superior vena cava obstruction.

> Rheumatoid arthritis – consider cricoarytenoid ankylosis.

Investigation

> **Hazard**
> If the patient has stridor and is in respiratory distress, then do not delay treatment and senior input while waiting for the results of investigations! Quick action to stabilise the airway and maintain adequate oxygenation is vital to prevent catastrophe.

If the patient is in a fit enough state to enable investigation, then the following are most likely to be helpful in revealing the diagnosis. Routine haematological and biochemical screening tests should also be performed:

> * Chest radiograph – may demonstrate evidence of underlying malignancy, mediastinal enlargement (lymphadenopathy/mediastinal tumour) or retrosternal thyroid. A lateral neck radiograph may also be informative.

> * Nasoendoscopy – the investigation of choice in a patient with unexplained stridor. It should be performed by an experienced operator with appropriate anaesthetic cover in the event of deterioration; and may demonstrate the presence of oedema, inflammation, foreign body, mucus plugging or tumour.

> * Bronchoscopy – enables visualisation of the trachea and bronchi, which may enable diagnosis and therapeutic intervention.

> * CT scan of the neck and thorax – may determine the level and cause of the obstruction, but not an investigation that can be performed without securing the airway if there is significant compromise.

> * Flow-volume loops – useful when the cause of breathlessness is not obvious to establish whether or not there is upper airway obstruction.

Management

> **Key point**
> In patients with life-threatening stridor the priority is to gain control of the airway – this may necessitate intubation or tracheotomy (to bypass upper airway obstruction) before any further intervention.

> **Key point**
> Treat the following conditions on suspicion:
>
> * Laryngeal oedema – give nebulised adrenaline (5 mL 1/1,000, neat) and high-dose steroids (ie 200 mg IV hydrocortisone or 8–16 mg IV dexamethasone).
>
> * Epiglottitis or laryngeal infection, or retropharyngeal abscess – give high-dose broad-spectrum intravenous antibiotics.

1.3.12 Pneumothorax

> **Case history**
> You are called to the emergency department to review a 28-year-old man complaining of breathlessness and chest pain. On your arrival he is tachypnoeic, with pulse oximetry showing SaO_2 93% on a FiO_2 of 60%. His girlfriend tells you that about 4 hours ago he complained of right-sided chest pain followed by progressive breathlessness. He is on no regular medication and is a lifelong non-smoker. A chest radiograph has just been done and confirms that he has a pneumothorax. How would you proceed?

Introduction

The first priority – as always – will be to make an assessment of the severity of illness, as described in Section 1.3.2, but the top priority in this case must clearly be to exclude tension pneumothorax.

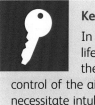

> **Key point**
> **Diagnosis of a tension pneumothorax:**
>
> > * the patient may be nearly dead
> > * cyanosis
> > * substantial respiratory effort – unless exhausted – but with little air movement
> > * chest looks 'blown up' on affected side
> > * tracheal deviation away from the affected side
> > * hyperresonance on percussion of the affected side
> > * absent breath sounds on the affected side.

> **Key point**
> **Treatment of a tension pneumothorax**
> **Do not delay if you suspect tension pneumothorax – treat immediately!**
> Put a hollow needle into the chest in the midaxillary line on the affected side above the level of the nipple.

History of the presenting problem

In this case the diagnosis is already established, but in a less dramatic presentation the following features would suggest a diagnosis of an acute spontaneous pneumothorax:

> * Nature of onset of the breathlessness – the patient is often able to pinpoint the exact time at which the

breathlessness started, with sudden onset often in association with unilateral pleuritic chest pain. Many patients, particularly those with primary pneumothoraces (no evidence of coexisting lung disease), do not seek medical advice for several days.

> Chest pain – pleuritic pain results from damage to the pleural surfaces, and in conjunction with reduced ventilatory units (collapsed lung) it can compromise gas exchange as a result of hypoventilation due to pain.

> Absence of fever or infective symptomatology – would argue against pneumonia being a cause of breathlessness and pleuritic chest pain.

Other relevant history

> Previous history of pneumothorax – the risk of recurrence of a primary pneumothorax is about 50% within the first 4 years, with risk factors including smoking, height in male patients and age over 60 years. Risk factors for recurrence of secondary pneumothoraces include age, pulmonary fibrosis and emphysema.

> Smoking history – the risk of developing a pneumothorax is increased in smokers, with a lifetime risk of 12% in men that smoke in comparison to 0.1% in male non-smokers. The same trend is seen in women although to a lesser extent. The risk of recurrence is also higher in those who continue to smoke.

> Coexistent lung disease – the presence of coexisting lung disease, ie COPD, will increase the risk of the development of a pneumothorax (secondary pneumothorax), but will also have implications in relation to the ability of the patient to tolerate the complication. A relatively small pneumothorax may cause significant respiratory compromise in a patient with pre-existing lung disease.

Examination

The first priority is to exclude the presence of a tension pneumothorax. The signs may not be dramatic in a pneumothorax that is not under tension, but look specifically for reduced expansion, breath sounds, tactile vocal fremitus and vocal resonance on the affected side in association with a hyperresonant percussion note.

Also note any signs of associated lung pathology (eg COPD), which would not be expected in this young man; or any other predisposing condition, eg Marfan syndrome.

Investigation

This man with an almost certain primary pneumothorax has already had the two key investigations: measurement of oxygen saturation and a chest radiograph (Fig 22). If the patient is very unwell or their SaO_2 is <92%, then ABGs should be checked to assess ventilation. In those with background lung disease, even a small pneumothorax may cause significant deterioration in oxygenation and hypercapnia.

When a pneumothorax is expected but not confirmed on the chest radiograph, or it is in the presence of severe

underlying emphysematous lung disease, then CT scanning is becoming an increasingly useful tool. It is vital that large bullae are not mistaken for a pneumothorax.

Key point

What is a 'large' and what is a 'small' pneumothorax?

BTS guidelines on pleural disease define as follows:

> Small – a visible rim of air of <2 cm between the lung and the chest-wall margin.

> Large – a visible rim of air >2 cm between the lung and the chest-wall margin.

Management

The appropriate management will depend on the size of the pneumothorax, the degree of respiratory compromise and whether or not the patient has underlying respiratory problems. For example:

> Small primary pneumothorax without significant breathlessness – observation alone is recommended. Patients with small primary

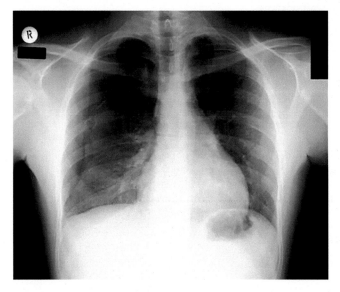

Fig 22 Large right-sided pneumothorax.

pneumothoraces and minimal symptoms do not require admission to hospital, but it should be stressed that in the event of developing any symptoms of breathlessness or chest pain they should return to hospital immediately.

> Small secondary pneumothorax without significant breathlessness – observation alone is appropriate in those with a pneumothorax <1 cm in depth, but hospitalisation is recommended in all cases.

Intervention is required for all patients with either primary or secondary pneumothoraces who are symptomatic, and in all patients with large pneumothoraces. All these patients require oxygen and adequate analgesia. Inhalation of a high concentration of oxygen increases the rate of resolution / air reabsorption fourfold every 24 hours. It is vitally important to maintain adequate analgesia to enable the patient to ventilate without pain and thus encourage re-expansion.

> Simple aspiration – this is recommended as first-line treatment for all primary pneumothoraces requiring intervention. In patients with secondary pneumothoraces it is only recommended as an initial treatment in small cases with minimal symptoms, and if treatment is successful it is recommended that these patients be observed in hospital for 24 hours prior to discharge.

> Intercostal chest drain – should be inserted if simple aspiration fails (see Section 3.5), and is recommended in most patients with secondary pneumothoraces. There is no evidence that large tubes (28–32 Fr) are any better than small tubes (12–14 Fr), so use a small bore tube initially – although this may have to be replaced with a larger tube if there is a persistent air leak.

Failure of a pneumothorax to re-expand after 24–48 hours requires specialist respiratory referral. High-pressure, low-volume suction (−5 to −15 cm water) may need to be considered. Surgical referral should be made at 3–5 days for those with a persistent air leak, and earlier in those with pre-existing lung disease who have a greater potential for complications.

Further comments

Patients discharged without intervention should be asked to reattend for a repeat chest radiograph in 10–14 days. In all other patients, resolution of the pneumothorax should be confirmed on a chest radiograph prior to discharge, with further follow up in 4–6 weeks.

The BTS Air Travel Working Party suggests that patients may travel safely by air 6 weeks after the resolution of a pneumothorax on chest radiography. There is still a significant risk of recurrence up to 1 year after resolution depending on whether the patient has an underlying lung disease or not, and because of this some patients may decide to avoid increasing the risk by not flying for a year.

Diving should be discouraged permanently after a pneumothorax unless a definitive surgical intervention has been performed.

1.3.13 Upper gastrointestinal haemorrhage

Case history

A 70-year-old woman is brought to hospital having collapsed in her home. On arrival of the ambulance she was hypotensive (BP 82/44 mmHg), cold and sweaty. The ambulance crew report that there was evidence that she had vomited blood at home, and that she did so again while en route. You are asked to assess her urgently.

Introduction

Key point

This woman is clearly extremely unwell: your first priority must be to initiate resuscitation (see Section 1.3.2). Only when resuscitation is underway should your attention move towards trying to work out the cause of her haematemesis.

History of the presenting problem

This woman is most unlikely to be able to give much of a history at the moment, but in a patient who was less ill the following information should be sought:

> Has she vomited blood before; and if so, what was the cause?

> Has she had a peptic ulcer in the past?

> Is there a history of heartburn, dyspepsia, use of medications for indigestion or previous barium meal / endoscopy that might point to peptic ulcer disease?

> What medications is she on? Enquire about both prescribed and 'over-the-counter' medications; take note of anticoagulants, NSAIDs and steroids in particular.

> Has she had liver disease in the past or is she at risk of this? After explaining why you need to know this information, ask in particular about their alcohol intake – 'Are you a heavy drinker now or have you ever been in the past?'

> Has there been recent weight loss, dysphagia or an early feeling of fullness when eating that might point to a malignancy?

Hazard

Are you sure the problem is haematemesis? In this case there does not seem to be any doubt, but patients often report that they have had 'dark vomit' and this might not be due to haematemesis. Keep an open mind to alternative diagnoses until haematemesis is proven, particularly intestinal obstruction, which commonly presents with vomitus that is interpreted as 'coffee-ground vomit' in the absence of any gastrointestinal bleeding at all.

Table 8	Physical signs in patients with liver disease	
Signs of chronic liver disease	**Signs of portal hypertension**	**Signs of hepatic encephalopathy**
Spider naevi	Splenomegaly	Myoclonic jerks – the 'liver flap'
Palmar erythema	Ascites	Hepatic foetor
Leuconychia	Caput medusae	Impaired conscious level
Clubbing (rarely)		
Jaundice		
Bruising		
Scratch marks		
Gynaecomastia		
Loss of secondary sexual hair		
Testicular atrophy		

Examination

The overall condition of the patient and the circulation should be assessed as described in Section 1.3.2, but with regard to someone with upper gastrointestinal bleeding note the following in addition:

> signs of chronic liver disease or portal hypertension (Table 8 and Fig 23)

> signs suggesting chronic iron-deficiency anaemia – pale conjunctivae, smooth tongue, angular stomatitis and koilonychia

> signs of malignancy – look for Virchow's node and/or an epigastric mass

> digital rectal examination – looking for melaena

> signs of aspiration.

Do not forget the rarities: finding subcutaneous emphysema in a patient with a history of severe vomiting is suggestive of Boerhaave syndrome (oesophageal rupture) and requires prompt consideration of surgical therapy; telangiectasia may indicate Osler–Weber–Rendu syndrome.

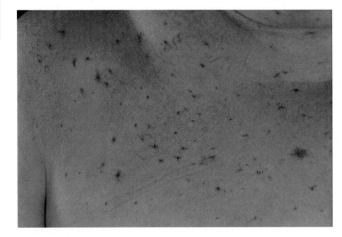

Fig 23 Spider naevi in a patient with alcohol-induced cirrhosis.

Investigation

Blood tests

This woman has clearly had a large bleed: arrange emergency cross match of 4 units of her blood; group and save them in a case without haemodynamic disturbance. FBC, clotting screen, electrolytes, and renal and liver function tests – remember that a relatively normal haemoglobin does not exclude significant haemorrhage because there may have been insufficient time for haemodilution to have taken place; and an iron-deficient picture suggests acute on chronic blood loss.

Other tests

Chest radiograph (portable; perform upright if the patient is very ill) if there is suspicion of aspiration. An abdominal film is extremely unlikely to provide diagnostic help in cases of gastrointestinal bleeding if there is no evidence of concomitant peritonism or intestinal obstruction: do not ask for one unless these are plausible diagnoses. An ECG to look for coronary ischaemia/infarction precipitated by hypotension.

Tests to determine the cause of bleeding

The definitive investigation for haematemesis, which can also be therapeutic, is upper gastrointestinal endoscopy (Fig 24). This should be performed after resuscitation of any patient who has had a significant haematemesis, or – in skilled hands – while resuscitation is ongoing in the patient who is continuing to bleed.

Hazard
It is not safe to endoscope a patient who is shocked and hypotensive.

Hazard
Remember that upper gastrointestinal bleeding in the setting of alcohol abuse is often caused by pathology other than oesophageal or gastric varices.

Management

Key point
Gastrointestinal bleeding is a team game – if haemorrhage is profuse, continuing or recurrent, then get a surgical opinion sooner rather than later.

The immediate priority is to resuscitate (see Section 1.3.1 and 1.3.2), but note in particular:

> Establish venous access – insert a large cannula into both antecubital fossae. If access is difficult, insert a line into the femoral vein (which lies medial to the artery, as remembered by the acronym 'NAVY' – Nerve, Artery, Vein and Y-fronts): if you cannot do this – get someone who can.

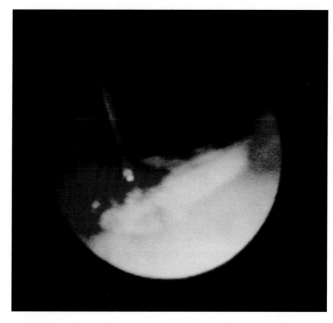

Fig 24 A photograph taken at endoscopy showing a peptic ulcer with a spurting artery – an obvious case for intervention.

Hazard
Never attempt central venous cannulation of a neck vein in a collapsed, hypovolaemic patient because the veins are constricted, rendering the procedure difficult. Insertion of a central line has never made anyone better, but it has killed.

> Give intravenous fluids – 1 L 0.9% saline as fast as possible while waiting for blood to arrive; then repeat the examination of pulse rate, BP and JVP. If hypotension persists and the JVP remains low, give more fluid rapidly (blood if available or 0.9% saline) until the JVP is raised to the upper limit of normal and postural hypotension is abolished.

> Insert urinary catheter (the poor man's central venous pressure (CVP)) – a good urine output is a much better marker of the restoration of organ perfusion than any CVP measurement.

> Proton pump inhibitors – omeprazole 80 mg IV bolus followed by infusion of 8 mg/h for 72 hours has been shown to reduce the early rebleed rate in peptic ulcer with haemorrhage.

Further comment

Risk scoring in upper gastrointestinal haemorrhage

Haematemesis is a more serious symptom than melaena – mortality rises from 5% in patients suffering melaena with clear nasogastric aspirate to 12% in those with melaena and fresh blood in the nasogastric aspirate; patients passing red blood per rectum with fresh blood in the nasogastric aspirate are reported to have a mortality rate of 29%; older patients have a higher mortality; and the mortality of all patients who rebleed in hospital is 40%.

A combination of clinical features and endoscopic findings has provided a numerical scoring system of risk in upper gastrointestinal haemorrhage (Table 9), the maximum additive score prior to diagnosis by endoscopy being 7.

Varices

Bleeding oesophageal varices can cause a torrential loss of blood. Get specialist help immediately if this is likely to be the diagnosis. Urgent endoscopy is mandatory – banding or sclerotherapy can be attempted during the procedure. Give terlipressin to reduce portal BP (2 mg IV, followed by 1 or 2 mg every 4–6 hours until bleeding is controlled, for up to 72 hours). Have a Sengstaken–Blakemore tube available, but this should only be used by those with experience of the technique. Patients with massive bleeding should be considered for intubation to reduce the increased risk of aspiration. Surgical treatment for acute variceal bleeding is rarely done because of high mortality, but the transjugular intrahepatic portosystemic shunt (TIPS) procedure can be considered in some cases. Patients should also be treated with empirical antibiotics which have been shown to improve survival in variceal bleeding.

1.3.14 Bloody diarrhoea

Case history

A 37-year-old woman is sent to the medical assessment unit by her GP with a 48-hour history of frequent watery diarrhoea which has subsequently become mixed with blood. Her bowels have opened 10 times over the past 24 hours. You are asked to review her.

History of the presenting problem

Intensity and nature of the diarrhoea

> Has the patient got diarrhoea at all? The history seems clear cut in this case, but patients use the term diarrhoea to describe different things. How many times have they opened their bowels today? Be aware that a sudden fall in stool frequency can indicate acute colonic dilatation and subsequent perforation.

> What is the nature of the diarrhoea? Frequent passage of small amounts of stool suggests proctitis or a rectal lesion; large volumes indicate small bowel pathology. Bloody diarrhoea is very suggestive of colonic pathology, whereas copious foul-smelling bulky stools that are difficult to flush away are characteristic of malabsorption.

> Is there diarrhoea at night? This is useful in distinguishing irritable bowel syndrome from organic pathology.

Key point

Physiology of the bowel

The daily dietary intake of food and liquid combined with gastric and intestinal secretions results in a volume load of about 7 L entering the small intestine. By the time intestinal contents have reached the terminal ileum only about 1.5 L remains, hence small bowel pathology often causes large-volume diarrhoea.

Precipitating factors

Consider infectious causes – has the patient eaten any food that they think may have been contaminated or infected? Has anyone else that they know had a similar problem? Have they been abroad recently? Clues to specific intestinal infections in the patient presenting with diarrhoea are shown in Table 10. Also ask about medication: have they taken antibiotics recently, which predispose to *Clostridium difficile*? Have they taken NSAIDs? These are a potent cause of colonic irritation and bloody diarrhoea.

Other relevant history

Has there been a previous history of bowel problems (could this be a flare of known inflammatory bowel disease?), bowel surgery or abdominal irradiation ('radiation colitis' can present with bloody diarrhoea). Is there any other relevant pathology? The sudden onset of pain and bloody diarrhoea in an older arteriopath should alert you to the possibility of ischaemic colitis.

The possibility of sexually transmitted infections and HIV-related infection must be considered if the diagnosis does not become apparent, in which case it will be necessary to take a sexual history. As always, this must be done with tact: explain why you need the information before asking for it and proceed carefully.

Examination

The overall condition of the patient and their circulation should be assessed as described in Section 1.3.2, but in someone with bloody diarrhoea take particular note of:

> General features – fever, nutritional status and anaemia.

> Abdomen – distension, peritonism, masses and character of bowel sounds.

> Digital rectal examination – inspect the perineum first, looking for skin changes or fistulae suggestive of Crohn's disease; palpate for a rectal mass; and examine any faeces for melaena or frank blood.

Investigations

Blood tests

Full blood count (FBC) – it may show acute anaemia, but it may also indicate chronic pathology, eg poorly controlled inflammatory bowel disease. The blood film and haematological indices are important – microcytic, hypochromic changes are likely to indicate blood loss, whereas macrocytosis points to malabsorption or alcohol abuse. A slight elevation in white cell count is of little help in differential diagnosis, but if the count is significantly elevated then do consider sepsis.

Electrolytes and renal/liver/bone profiles – severe diarrhoea can cause profound hypokalaemia; and a serum albumin of <30 g/L is a bad feature in inflammatory bowel disease because albumin loss is proportional to the extent of bowel involvement. An elevated CRP may indicate significant inflammation or infection.

Cultures

Faeces should be sent for microbiological investigation (microscopy, culture and specific testing for *Clostridium difficile* toxin) and the sample can be obtained during sigmoidoscopy if the patient has not opened their bowels before this is performed. Also send blood cultures.

Table 10	Clues to particular intestinal infections	
Site of infection	**Infectious agent**	**Predisposing cause**
Small bowel infection	Cholera	Foreign travel
	Enterotoxigenic *Escherichia coli*	Infected meat
	Rotavirus Norovirus (*Norwalk virus*) Small round virus	Common and associated with vomiting
	Toxin-producing *Staphylococcus aureus*	Symptoms a few hours after ingestion of contaminated material; associated with vomiting
	Toxin-producing *Bacillus cereus*	Classically associated with contaminated rice and accompanied by vomiting
	Campylobacter jejuni	Commonest infectious cause in the UK today; beware of undercooked chicken
Colonic infection	*Shigella* and *Salmonella*	Classical cause of dysentery and associated with bloody diarrhoea
	Amoebiasis	Can be contracted in UK, so an important consideration on acute medical 'intake'
	Clostridium difficile	Associated with antibiotic therapy; toxin-producing
	Enterohaemorrhagic *Escherichia coli*	Produces a Shiga-like toxin; can cause haemolytic uraemic syndrome

Radiology

An erect chest radiograph should include the hemidiaphragms to look for evidence of perforation (Fig 25). A supine abdominal film should be taken to exclude toxic dilatation and to look for mucosal islands and a dilated small bowel, which are other adverse prognostic radiological signs of inflammatory bowel disease (Fig 26).

Sigmoidoscopy

Sigmoidoscopy (Fig 27) should be performed after the abdominal radiograph because introduction of air during the procedure can produce a picture alarmingly similar to toxic dilatation. Normal rectal mucosa usually excludes active ulcerative colitis. Inflamed rectal mucosa can be a feature of any cause of severe diarrhoea. The mucosal appearance of *Clostridium difficile* infection is also variable, although the adherent yellow-white plaques, or 'pseudomembrane', is characteristic. A rectal biopsy should be taken below the peritoneal reflection, ie within 10 cm of the anal margin.

Key point

Findings of concern in acute ulcerative colitis:

> bowels open 9–12 times in the first 24 hours

> pulse >100 beats per minute

> fever >38°C

> albumin <30 g/L

> CRP >45 mg/L

> mucosal islands, toxic megacolon and dilated small bowel on abdominal radiograph.

Management

Resuscitation, if required, will as always be the immediate priority (see Section 1.3.2). Specific

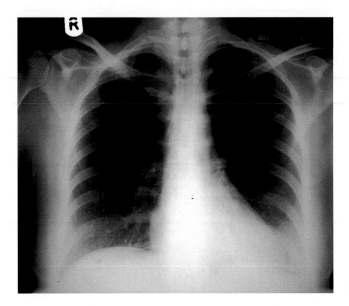

Fig 25 Chest radiograph showing air under both hemidiaphragms. No apologies for the subtle changes – they are often as subtle in real life!

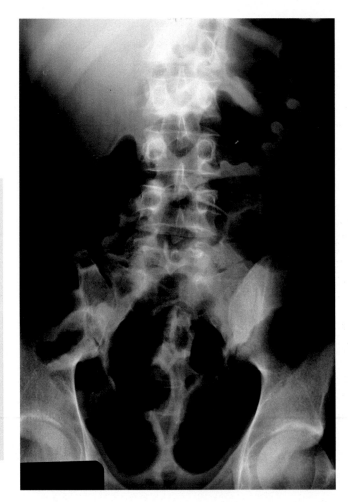

Fig 26 Abdominal radiograph in acute ulcerative colitis. The colon is dilated (not quite to 10 cm, but worrying nonetheless). Thumbprinting of colonic mucosa is seen in the left upper abdomen and there are dilated loops of the small bowel.

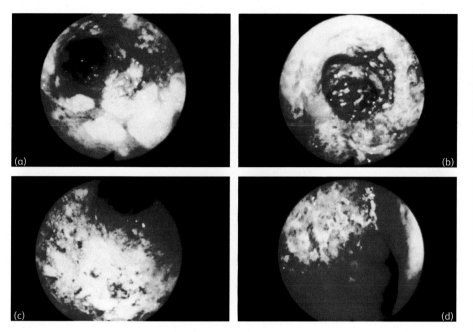

Fig 27 Sigmoidoscopic appearances of ulcerative colitis, showing inflamed mucosa, ulceration and contact bleeding.

management will depend on the cause of the problem, but note the following:

> Infective colitis – must be considered in all cases of acute colitis. If the patient is very ill and you cannot exclude infection, then it is safer to treat empirically with a combination of ciprofloxacin and metronidazole (but follow local guidelines). This will cover most potential pathogens, including amoebae and *Clostridium difficile*.

> Pseudomembranous colitis – associated with antibiotic usage, particularly third-generation cephalosporins. Treat with metronidazole (IV or PO) and/or vancomycin (PO) after sigmoidoscopy (and rectal biopsy) has been performed and stool has been sent for *Clostridium difficile* toxin.

> Inflammatory bowel disease – a moderate or severe exacerbation

should be treated with systemic steroids (eg methylprednisolone 40 mg IV bd) and rectal steroid enemas. Less severe exacerbations (perhaps limited to the rectum) may be appropriately managed with rectal steroid preparations, with or without oral or intravenous steroids. 5-aminosalicylic acid products may also have a role. Other immunological agents (eg infliximab, ciclosporin) may be required in some severe cases.

 Hazard

In patients with known inflammatory bowel disease, early involvement of the colorectal surgical team is mandatory: do not wait until there is radiographic evidence of toxic megacolon or perforation.

1.3.15 Abdominal pain

 Case history

A 42-year-old woman is referred to the emergency department with epigastric and back pain that has progressively worsened over the preceding 48 hours. She has been unable to eat for the last 24 hours because of nausea and vomiting, and she is in significant discomfort. The 'on-call' surgeon has seen her and said that 'the problem is not surgical', hence she has been referred to the medical team and you are asked to assess her.

Introduction

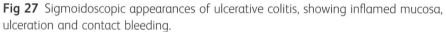 **Key point**

Patients do not know whether their abdominal pain is 'surgical' or 'medical' – as a physician you must be wary of the acute abdomen that has been incorrectly referred, those conditions that may require joint management (eg biliary tract diseases), and the rare medical mimics of a 'surgical abdomen' (basal pneumonia, atypical presentation of MI, diabetic ketoacidosis (DKA), shingles before the rash, and porphyria).

History of the presenting problem

Onset and time course of pain

Most cases of abdominal pain start gradually, but perforation of a viscus can occasionally cause sudden pain. The pain of duodenal ulceration is typically severe in the early hours of the morning, and there may be a definite periodicity to the pain, ie nightly bouts of pain for a few weeks followed by a symptom-free period. Severe acute pain persisting for several hours often implies a catastrophic event such as perforation, strangulation or intestinal obstruction.

Biliary pain often becomes more intense with time, but can be relieved suddenly with the passage of a stone.

Precipitating or relieving factors

Pain from the parietal peritoneum is exacerbated by even slight movement, which explains why patients with peritonitis lie perfectly still. By contrast, visceral pain often causes the patient to writhe around in an attempt to find a more comfortable position when a spasm of pain attacks.

Relief of pain by food is a strong pointer to peptic ulceration. Exacerbation by food implies an obstructive component, gastritis or oesophagitis. Gastric or duodenal inflammation is associated with alcohol, aspirin and other NSAIDs. Diffuse abdominal pain appearing 2 minutes to 1 hour after a meal raises the possibility of intestinal angina (mesenteric ischaemia). Oesophageal pain is typically brought on by bending or stooping. Pain which is aggravated by tension or anxiety is a feature of irritable bowel syndrome.

Nature and distribution of pain

Constant, generalised and severe pain that is exacerbated by any movement is highly suggestive of peritonitis. Colicky pain is likely to be visceral in origin. The site where visceral pain is experienced depends on the intestinal segment involved: oesophageal pain is often in the epigastrium or low central chest; duodenal pain is felt in the epigastrium or just to the right of it; small bowel pain is poorly localised and is generally felt diffusely in the periumbilical region; and colonic pain usually occurs in roughly the area of the diseased colonic segment. Pain that is maximal in the right upper quadrant points to biliary tract disease, and pain sited in the flank with radiation to the anterior abdomen and inguinal region is suggestive of renal colic. Pancreatic pain is sited in the epigastrium, but there is often a lot of associated discomfort in the lumbar region of the back; pancreatitis is also a potential cause of generalised abdominal pain, which can mimic the peritonism of a ruptured viscus.

Hazard

Patients must not be denied analgesia, but once this has been given the nature and distribution of pain may change dramatically.

Referral of pain

Pain may be referred from visceral organs or the parietal peritoneum to areas innervated by the same dermatome: oesophageal pain may radiate to the neck and arms; gall bladder pain radiates to the right infrascapular region, where there may be hyperaesthesia over the referred area; and pain from a duodenal ulcer that radiates through to the back usually indicates penetration of the ulcer into the pancreas.

!

Hazard

Be wary of thoracic pathology masquerading as an acute abdomen – pleurisy of the lower pleural surfaces can result in referred pain in the upper abdomen.

Associated symptoms

A full functional enquiry related to the abdomen is clearly required. This woman has been vomiting – how often, what, how much and does it relieve the pain? How are her bowels? Have these been normal, when was the last bowel motion and was it normal? Has she had any urinary symptoms – frequency, dysuria, haematuria and pneumaturia? When was her last period, and was it normal? Has she been feverish? And as a marker of longer standing illness, has she lost any weight recently?

Other relevant history

> Drug history – codeine- or morphine-based drugs predispose to constipation with or without subacute obstruction. NSAIDs predispose to peptic ulceration. Oral contraceptives may increase the risk of gallstone formation.

> Alcohol – acute abdominal pain in alcoholics may result from gastritis, peptic ulceration, acute pancreatitis, tense ascites or spontaneous bacterial peritonitis.

> Past medical history – always ask if there is any history of similar presentations, and if so what diagnosis has been established (if any). Previous abdominal operations raise the possibility of adhesions that can cause intestinal

obstruction. Comorbid illnesses may also be relevant in both diagnosis (eg the patient with widespread arterial disease is more likely to have an ischaemic gut) and in assessing the fitness of the patient for surgery (should it be a management option).

Examination

The overall condition of the patient and their circulation should be assessed as described in Section 1.3.2, but in someone with acute abdominal pain note the following in particular:

> Inspection – how does the patient appear? Unwell, in pain, lying still or writhing around? Are they holding their abdomen rigidly? Is the abdomen distended, or are there any obvious masses? Is there any bruising of the body wall that may occur with pancreatitis, ie umbilical (Cullen's sign) or in the flanks (Grey Turner's sign)?

> Palpation – is there peritonism? Are there localised abdominal findings, eg local tenderness with or without a mass, an enlarged organ, or perhaps a pyonephrosis or an empyema of the gall bladder? Always examine the hernial orifices, remembering to look carefully in 'unusual sites', eg periumbilical.

> Auscultation – are the bowel sounds normal or do they sound obstructed? Is there complete silence suggesting peritonitis?

> Digital rectal examination – this may reveal hard stool in the older, compacted and obstructed patient; or the rectum may be empty as in small bowel obstruction. Tenderness in the right iliac fossa on rectal examination is common in patients with appendicitis.

Look specifically for cachexia and/or enlarged supraclavicular lymph nodes, suggesting malignancy; and also for evidence of chronic liver disease (see Section 1.3.13).

Investigation

Key point

The patient with obvious peritonism requires immediate resuscitation, analgesia, urgent surgical review and a laparotomy.

Blood tests

> Full blood count (FBC) – anaemia may indicate chronic gastrointestinal blood loss; elevated white cell count may be due to pancreatitis.

> Urea and electrolytes (U&E) – look for hypokalaemia due to vomiting, renal impairment, raised urea in upper gastrointestinal blood loss and/or dehydration.

> Liver function tests (LFTs) and bone profile – an abnormal liver profile may indicate a biliary cause for the presentation; and elevated serum calcium may in rare cases explain the patient's abdominal pain.

> Amylase – must be checked without fail: a raised serum amylase can be seen in acute cholecystitis and in peptic ulceration, but if the serum amylase is five times greater than normal then pancreatitis is likely.

> C-reactive protein (CRP), which will be non-specific if raised but reassuring if normal.

> Blood glucose – acute diabetic ketoacidosis (DKA) can present with abdominal pain.

Imaging

> Erect chest X-ray – better at diagnosing perforation than an abdominal film and may also show unexpected lower lobe pathology

(pneumonia or collapse due to splinting of the diaphragm).

> Supine abdominal radiograph – may diagnose intestinal obstruction or help to localise pathology, eg the dilated contiguous loop of bowel in cholecystitis, the pattern of bowel dilatation seen with sigmoid volvulus or the classical appearances of toxic megacolon. Look for biliary or renal stones. Is there pancreatic calcification suggestive of previous pancreatitis?

> Abdominal ultrasonography – helpful if you suspect biliary disease.

> Abdominal CT scan – useful in identifying intestinal obstruction; perforation and likely source; pancreatitis (Fig 28).

Other investigations

If there is a clinical suspicion of infection, send blood cultures, urine cultures and stool cultures. An arterial or venous blood gas is also useful if patients appear unwell – look for metabolic acidosis and raised lactate.

Management

Key point

The on-call surgeon has said that this patient does not have a 'surgical abdomen' – but if you disagree, talk with him or her and get a senior review.

Resuscitation, if required, will as always be the immediate priority (see Section 1.3.2). Specific management will depend on the cause of the problem, but note:

> Nil by mouth with or without a nasogastric tube – a nasogastric tube should be placed to clear the stomach contents if the patient continues to vomit or there is evidence of obstruction; and the patient should remain nil by mouth until a diagnosis and management plan have been formulated.

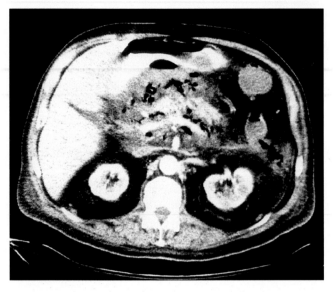

Fig 28 CT scan showing necrotising pancreatitis with gas formation. The patient had presented with abdominal pain indistinguishable from that due to peritonitis.

> Urinary catheter – close monitoring of urine output is essential in any patient who is critically unwell.

> Antibiotics – if there is evidence of sepsis then broad-spectrum antibiotics should be given promptly after cultures have been taken, guided by microbiological advice and local policy.

Further comments

Very rare causes of an acute abdomen include:

> Acute intermittent porphyria – an inborn error of the synthesis of haem, resulting in overproduction of the intermediate compounds called porphyrins. Commonly presents around 30 years of age with abdominal pain, vomiting and constipation.

> Diabetic ketoacidosis (DKA).

> Sickle cell crisis – vaso-occlusive problems may occur in the small vessels of any organs including the spleen, liver, kidneys and bowel.

> Familial Mediterranean fever – characterised by recurrent attacks of fever, arthritis and abdominal or chest pain.

1.3.16 Hepatic encephalopathy/ alcohol withdrawal

Case history

A 65-year-old woman is brought to the emergency department having been found confused and shaking in her flat. She is known to be an alcoholic and attends the emergency department regularly. Her warden told the ambulance crew that she had been vomiting recently.

Introduction

Your main concern in an alcoholic patient who presents with confusion and tremor is to exclude any serious or life-threatening condition. Do not assume that the patient is just drunk – this is a dangerous thing to do, both for you and for the patient. Consider the differential diagnosis shown in Table 11 as you gather the history.

History of the presenting problem

Key point

When dealing with a 'confused' patient:

> Make sure the problem is confusion and not dysarthria or dysphasia.

> Establish baseline GCS score (Fig 29).

> Establish baseline Abbreviated Mental Test Score.

Hazard

If you cannot get a history from the patient, you must try to get one from somebody else.

Key point

The Abbreviated Mental Test Score

Each question scores one mark, with a score of 6 or less out of 10 likely to indicate impaired cognition:

1) Patient's age.

2) What is the time, to the nearest hour?

3) Address – 42 West Street – to recall at the end of the test.

4) What year is it?

5) What is the name of this place?

6) Recognition of two people – can the patient recognise your job and that of a nurse?

7) Date of birth, day and month.

8) Year World War 2 began.

9) Name of present monarch/ prime minister.

10) Count backwards from 20 to 1.

Table 11 Differential diagnosis of confusion in an alcoholic	
Cause	Condition
Specifically alcohol related	Alcohol intoxication Acute alcohol withdrawal Delirium tremens Wernicke's encephalopathy
Acute on chronic liver failure	Hypoglycaemia Hepatic encephalopathy
Other cerebral	Subdural haematoma Postictal
Other	Any severe illness, particularly sepsis Hypothermia

Glasgow Coma Scale

Best eye opening response	Score
Spontaneously	4
To speech	3
To pain	2
None	1

Best verbal response	
Orientated	5
Confused conversation	4
Words	3
Sounds	2
None	1

Best motor response	
Obeys commands	6
Localisation to painful stimuli	5
Withdraws to pain	4
Flexor (decorticate) response to pain	3
Extensor (decerebrate) response to pain	2
No response	1

Notes
- Maximum score is 15, minimum is 3; coma is defined as 8 or less; significant deterioration is defined as a decrease in GCS score of 2 or more. Record components separately, eg patient with GCS 8 may be E2, V2, M4.
- Motor response should be scored as the best response of any limb.
- Painful stimuli – do not use methods that might lead to bleeding or bruising: the best techniques are to apply pressure to a nail bed by squeezing a pencil or biro hard against it, and rubbing the sternum hard with your knuckles.

Fig 29 Glasgow Coma Scale (GCS).

This woman will not be able to give a reliable history, but ask questions of anyone who knows anything about her circumstances and explore factors that may precipitate acute deterioration in someone with known alcoholic liver disease (if there are none, call the warden to try and get further details):

> Binge drinking or acute alcohol withdrawal – how much alcohol does she usually drink? Has she stopped over the past few days, or has she been on a 'bender' – an extended drinking session that has become so excessive she is no longer able to function?

> Gastrointestinal disturbance – a gastrointestinal bleed may cause acute decompensation, as may constipation.

> Trauma/head injury – alcoholics frequently fall over.

> Infection – any infection may cause deterioration. Ask particularly about respiratory or urinary symptoms and consider spontaneous bacterial peritonitis if ascites present.

> Drug history – a wide range of drugs can cause liver problems, but note especially those that commonly cause decompensation of chronic liver disease, eg analgesics, benzodiazepines, opioids and diuretics.

Examination

Begin with an overall assessment as described in Section 1.3.2 before proceeding to note the following:

General features

> Smell – does she smell of alcohol or is there a hepatic foetor?

> Evidence of hepatic encephalopathy – liver flap, and grade severity as shown in Table 12.

> Signs of chronic liver disease – see Section 1.3.13 and Fig 30.

> Nutritional status.

Abdominal

Examine for tenderness, hepatomegaly (unlikely in chronic liver disease), splenomegaly and ascites. Rectal examination for melaena is essential.

Key point

Abdominal tenderness can be the first sign of spontaneous bacterial peritonitis in a patient with chronic liver disease.

Table 12	Grades of hepatic encephalopathy
Grade	Status
1	Mildly drowsy but coherent; mood change, impaired concentration and psychomotor function
2	Drowsy and confused, but able to answer questions
3	Very drowsy but rousable; alternatively incoherent and agitated
4a	Responsive only to painful stimuli
4b	Unresponsive

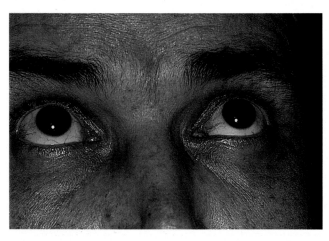

Fig 30 Always look carefully for jaundice. (Reproduced with permission: Axford J. *Medicine*. Oxford: Blackwell Science, 1996.)

Neurological

Aside from features of hepatic encephalopathy, look specifically for evidence of:

> Head injury/subdural haemorrhage – the risk of a subdural or extradural haematoma is high if the pupils are unequal or there are localising signs.

> Wernicke's encephalopathy.

> Korsakoff syndrome – gross defect of memory for recent events, with gaps in memory filled by confabulation.

Key point
Wernicke's encephalopathy

Look for the triad of:

> ophthalmoplegia – horizontal and/or vertical nystagmus; weakness/failure of eye abduction; and weakness/failure of conjugate gaze

> ataxia

> confusion.

Investigation

Key point

Check finger-prick blood glucose to exclude hypoglycaemia.

Routine blood tests

Full blood count (FBC), coagulation screen, electrolytes, renal/liver/bone profiles, glucose and an inflammatory marker (CRP) – a wide range of abnormalities may be found.

Tests to look for infection

Blood and urine cultures. Chest radiograph for signs of consolidation (check also for fractured ribs). If ascites is present then tap to look for evidence of spontaneous bacterial peritonitis, which is diagnosed if this reveals a neutrophil count $>500 \times 10^6$/L.

Other investigations

Depending on the clinical context it may be appropriate to check serum amylase or ammonia, perform ABGs, or organise a CT scan of the brain.

Management

Hazard

If there is a history of chronic alcohol intake or malnourishment, give thiamine IV before glucose to avoid precipitating Wernicke's encephalopathy. This is usually done by giving high-potency thiamine (Pabrinex); two pairs of ampoules IV.

Specific management will clearly depend on the diagnosis (Table 11), but if the working diagnosis is acute on chronic liver failure related to alcohol, then note the following.

Management of acute on chronic liver failure

Hypovolaemia and electrolyte disturbance

Treat abnormalities as follows:

> Hypoglycaemia – give intravenous glucose to maintain finger-prick blood glucose >3.5 mmol/L (the patient may also require continuous infusion of 10% dextrose) but only after giving thiamine.

> Hypovolaemia – give colloid (albumin) rather than the usual 0.9% saline.

> Hyponatraemia – this is common and is due to water excess, not sodium deficiency; hence treat with water restriction and not with 0.9% saline.

> Hypokalaemia – give intravenous potassium.

> Hypophosphataemia – start intravenous or oral replacement therapy.

Feeding and gastric protection

Nasogastric tube – adequate nutrition is important and drugs can be given reliably by this route. Ranitidine 50 mg IV three times daily – to reduce the risk of stress ulceration.

Reduction of intestinal nitrogenous load

Start lactulose 20–30 mL or lactitol 10 g three times daily, reducing the dose when diarrhoea starts; give a phosphate enema; and consider starting intravenous antibiotics if the patient is poorly responsive or comatose. Rifaximin can then be used to prevent further episodes of encephalopathy.

Coagulopathy

Give vitamin K orally or intravenously (preferable), and consider giving fresh frozen plasma or platelets if the patient is actively bleeding.

Underlying infection

Start broad-spectrum antibiotics (eg intravenous piperacillin/tazobactam 4.5 g four times daily or as per local protocol) if infection is suspected. Remember that bacterial peritonitis occurs in around 25% of patients with cirrhotic ascites.

Vitamin supplementation

Vitamins B and C are usually deficient in chronic alcoholics. Initially give thiamine (Pabrinex) IV 2–3 pairs eight-hourly (this can cause anaphylaxis). If the patient can take oral medications then follow with oral thiamine (50 mg od), vitamin B compound tablets strong (1–2 tablets tds) and vitamin C (100 mg od).

Anticipate and treat complications

Key point
The development of complications means a very poor prognosis and it may be inappropriate to 'escalate treatment'. This is an issue that requires careful consideration and discussion with senior colleagues. If in doubt, contact the regional liver centre for advice.

Acute kidney injury is a common complication of liver failure. It is most frequently due to acute tubular necrosis, although the prognosis for hepatorenal syndrome is particularly poor. Cerebral oedema is another feared complication: consider giving mannitol 200 mg/kg IV slowly; intracranial pressure monitoring can be useful but is not available in all centres.

Acute alcohol withdrawal and delirium tremens

Key point

Acute alcohol withdrawal
This is common; it typically causes tremor and confusion after 8–24 hours and settles after 48 hours.

Delirium tremens

This is rare, but can be fatal if untreated. Symptoms include tremor, confusion, visual hallucinations, fever and sweating; usually occurs 3–4 days after stopping drinking.

Aside from the standard supportive measures give vitamins (as above), treat hypoglycaemia and prescribe sedation:

> If the patient can tolerate oral therapy – give chlordiazepoxide 30 mg four times on day one, then treat with a reducing dose. Or, if appropriately trained staff are available, use a symptom-triggered dosing regimen utilising an assessment tool, such as the Clinical Institute Withdrawal Assessment of Alcohol, Revised (CIWA-Ar) scale.

> For patients who are severely agitated and unable to take oral medications then clomethiazole IV is an alternative option, although this is now rarely used. It can lead to fatal respiratory depression (especially in alcoholics with cirrhosis) and therefore close monitoring and full resuscitation facilities are essential.

1.3.17 Acute kidney injury, fluid overload and hyperkalaemia

Case history

A 67-year-old man had an elective hip replacement 5 days ago. Over the last 24 hours he has become increasingly breathless and the observation charts show that no urine output has been recorded, which the nurse in charge of the ward confirms to be true. The orthopaedic doctor on duty asks for an urgent medical review.

Introduction

The most likely explanation for this scenario is the development of postoperative acute kidney injury, and the most pressing concerns are that the patient might have hyperkalaemia and/or pulmonary oedema.

Key point

Hyperkalaemia can kill suddenly and without warning.

Recognition of significant hyperkalaemia

A 12-lead ECG should be done in all acutely unwell patients: in this case this might reveal changes diagnostic of MI or consistent with pulmonary embolism (PE), but the most important matter is to look for evidence of hyperkalaemia. The following ECG changes occur sequentially as the patient's serum potassium rises:

> tall 'peaked' T-waves

> flattened P-waves; prolonged P-R interval; and wide QRS complexes

> absent P-waves; very wide QRS complexes slurring into T-waves (Fig 31)

> cardiac arrest – VF, VT and asystole.

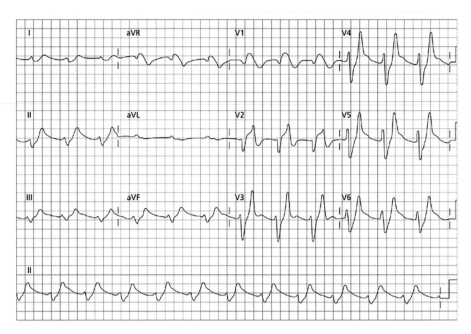

Fig 31 ECG changes in severe hyperkalaemia.

Urgent treatment is required if there is any change more severe than T-wave peaking; take a specimen for measurement of the serum potassium, but do not wait for the result! It is not a triumph to be told that the serum potassium was 9.1 mmol/L just after the patient has arrested.

Treatment of significant hyperkalaemia

If the patient's ECG looks like that in Fig 31 then give calcium gluconate immediately, followed by dextrose/insulin or salbutamol:

> Calcium gluconate, 10% solution, 10 mL IV over 1–2 minutes – this does not lower the serum potassium level but reduces myocardial excitability. Its effect is instant, with the ECG becoming less abnormal in front of your eyes.

> Dextrose – 50% solution, 50 mL – with 10 U short-acting insulin (eg Actrapid (soluble insulin)) IV over 15–30 minutes. This shifts potassium into the intracellular compartment. It should not cause hypoglycaemia, but check finger-prick blood glucose if in any doubt. Serum potassium falls by 1–2 mmol/L over 30–60 minutes.

> Salbutamol 10 mg, nebulised – this activates the intracellular adenylate cyclase system and induces a shift of potassium into the intracellular compartment. Serum potassium falls by 1–2 mmol/L over 30–60 minutes.

Key point

Calcium, dextrose/insulin and salbutamol are holding measures only, reducing the serum potassium concentration for 4–6 hours. Most patients with severe hyperkalaemia require urgent haemodialysis, the exceptions being the few whose renal function improves rapidly, eg after relief of acute obstruction.

After giving emergency treatment for hyperkalaemia, do not forget to contact the ICU or local renal unit to arrange transfer for urgent haemofiltration or dialysis if the patient's urine output does not respond immediately and dramatically to fluid and/or bladder catheterisation.

> **!** **Hazard**
> Oral or rectal ion exchange resins (eg calcium resonium) increase gut excretion of potassium but take 24 hours to have any effect and are not an emergency treatment for hyperkalaemia.

History of the presenting problem

After considering and (if necessary) treating hyperkalaemia, consider causes of breathlessness as described in Section 1.2.4 and find out from the patient, medical records and/or observation charts if he has any history of renal/urinary problems (any symptoms of prostatism?) or pre-existing renal impairment (what was the preoperative serum creatinine?). Investigate precisely what happened to him during his operation and afterwards, noting vital signs (was he hypotensive at any time, which might explain acute tubular necrosis?), daily fluid input/output, administration of drugs and whether he now feels as though he wants to pass urine (acute retention).

Examination

Is this man ill, very ill or nearly dead? As always, begin with an overall assessment as described in Section 1.3.2, taking particular care to look for evidence of the following.

Assessment of volume status

Given that the patient is anuric it is vital to assess their fluid status. Are they hypovolaemic or already fluid overloaded? Patients who are hypovolaemic may be hypotensive and tachycardic with cool peripheries, prolonged capillary refill time and dry mucus membranes. Patients who are fluid overloaded and have developed pulmonary oedema are likely to be breathless with tachypnoea. The JVP is likely to be raised and BP may be elevated. Listen to the heart sounds for a gallop rhythm indicating that the left ventricle is under strain. On auscultation of the chest are there bilateral crackles suggesting fluid overload?

Urinary retention

Is the bladder palpable?

Investigation

As described in Section 1.2.4, with the following of particular note in addition to the ECG:

> Electrolytes and renal function tests – to confirm the presence of hyperkalaemia and/or acute kidney injury. Acute kidney injury is defined as a rise in creatinine to 1.5X the baseline level or 6 hours of oliguria (urine output <0.5 mL/kg/h). Patients with acute kidney injury should have their electrolytes checked twice daily initially.

> Consider sepsis – a common precipitant of postoperative renal failure; take relevant cultures.

> Chest radiograph – looking at the heart size, and for pulmonary oedema or infection.

> ABGs – expecting a partially compensated metabolic acidosis in a sick patient with renal failure. A normal $PaCO_2$ would probably be worrying in this case as it would indicate that the patient is getting tired and losing respiratory compensation, in which case acidosis can worsen very rapidly.

> Ultrasound scan (USS) to exclude hydronephrosis.

> Urine dipstick to look for proteinuria.

Management

If this man looks very ill or about to die, then call for help from ICU immediately. Otherwise, proceed as described in Section 1.3.2 and take particular care to:

> Insert a urinary catheter – this will relieve outflow obstruction if it is present, which may result in a prompt diuresis and restoration of renal function.

> Stop nephrotoxins – NSAIDs (commonly used for postoperative analgesia), angiotensin-converting enzyme (ACE) inhibitors and angiotensin receptor blockers all have adverse effects on renal blood flow in this context and should be (temporarily) stopped, as should aminoglycoside antibiotics. If the patient is hypotensive then ensure other antihypertensives are also stopped.

> Commence intravenous fluids if patient is hypovolaemic. It is important to monitor the electrolytes and urine output regularly so that the rate and type of fluid can be adjusted appropriately.

Management of fluid overload in the patient with renal failure

> Sit the patient up.

> Give high-flow oxygen.

> Restrict fluid input to the minimum possible.

> Nitrate, eg isosorbide dinitrate 2–20 mg/h IV, titrated to as high a dose as the BP will allow.

> Diuretic, eg furosemide (frusemide) 250 mg IV over 1 hour, may induce some increase in urine output.

> Dialysis/ultrafiltration – arrange urgently if the patient has fluid overload which is not responsive to diuretics.

> Continuous positive airway pressure (CPAP) – can be very effective in treating breathlessness due to pulmonary oedema.

Hazard

When inserting a central line for dialysis access in a patient with pulmonary oedema:

> Do not lie the patient down to put one in – they are likely to arrest.

> Do not use the subclavian vein – the patient will not tolerate a pneumothorax.

> Use the femoral vein.

Key point

In acute kidney injury, renal replacement therapy (haemodialysis or haemofiltration) should be considered if any of the following are present:

> hyperkalaemia

> severe metabolic acidosis

> diuretic-resistant pulmonary oedema

> symptomatic uraemia, eg altered mental status, fits, asterixis and pericarditis.

Further comments

Patients undergoing surgery are exposed to a variety of factors that put them at risk of developing acute kidney injury:

> underlying illness leading to surgery (eg acute abdomen)

> perioperative hypotension

> reduced oral intake around the time of surgery

> nephrotoxic drugs eg intravenous contrast, aminoglycosides

> pain and opiates may lead to urinary retention.

The risk of acute kidney injury can be reduced by discontinuing nephrotoxic medications on admission, regular monitoring of BP, urine output and electrolytes, and trying to avoid periods of hypotension and oliguria.

1.3.18 Diabetic ketoacidosis

Case history

A 24-year-old student is brought to the emergency department by her boyfriend. He tells you that she has been unwell for 3 days and unable to attend lectures. She is a known diabetic and has had difficulty keeping liquids down for 24 hours because she has been vomiting. A finger-prick blood glucose has shown a reading of 'over 25 mmol/L'.

Introduction

Hazard

Patients with diabetes, like those with asthma, are used to managing their disease and are often extremely ill by the time they are willing to go to hospital.

History of presenting complaint

Duration of symptoms

How long has she been unwell? Diabetic ketoacidosis (DKA) typically develops over a few days with symptoms including nausea, vomiting, myalgia, headache and abdominal pain.

Evidence of infection

The stress of intercurrent illness is a common cause of loss of diabetic control, interrupted insulin therapy and resultant complications such as DKA. Pursue possible sources of infection –

respiratory, urinary, gastrointestinal and skin (ulcers and abscesses) are commonest; septicaemia and meningitis are less likely.

Recent monitoring and management of diabetes

What monitoring of her diabetes has the patient performed over the last few days, and what does this reveal? The first common error is for a diabetic to neglect the monitoring of blood glucose when they feel unwell. If monitoring has been performed, this may show evidence of worsening control with progressive hyperglycaemia over the duration of symptom deterioration. The second common error is for the diabetic who is unwell to omit taking any insulin because they are unable to eat. Simple poor compliance with insulin therapy can also ultimately result in DKA. Some patients will admit to this, but most often it is information from family or friends, or scrutiny of previous accounts in the medical notes that raises this suspicion.

Hazard

The two commonest errors of the sick diabetic:

> 'I was feeling too unwell to check my blood sugar'.

> 'I wasn't eating, so I didn't think I needed to take any insulin'.

Other relevant history

Duration and complications of diabetes

It will clearly be necessary to establish the duration of diabetes and whether or not the patient has suffered macrovascular complications, eg ischaemic heart disease, cerebrovascular disease and peripheral vascular disease, or microvascular complications, eg neuropathy, nephropathy and retinopathy. Hopefully she will not have done by the age of 24 years, but if she has had diabetes for 20 years then it is possible. However, this can wait until the next day once resuscitation is complete and the patient is feeling better.

Usual diabetic control

Preceding admissions with DKA or hypoglycaemia would suggest poor diabetic control, poor compliance and lack of education. If there have been previous presentations, is there a pattern to them and is there a common precipitating factor? What has been the HbA1c level?

Examination

The immediate priority, as always, will be to check 'ABC' (airway, breathing and circulation) and determine whether the patient is ill, very ill or nearly dead, with details of further assessment as described in Section 1.3.2. The following would be particularly important aspects in this case:

> Respiratory pattern and breath – has the patient got the sighing respiratory pattern of Kussmaul breathing induced by acidosis? The smell of ketones on the breath of the patient with DKA may make the diagnosis clear, but not everybody can smell them.

> Assessment of fluid status – patients with DKA are always very volume deplete. In addition to intravascular depletion (postural hypotension, postural tachycardia and low JVP) they are short of interstitial and intracellular fluid (dry mucous membranes, dry axillae, reduced skin turgor and sunken eyes).

> Sources of infection – it is important to consider all sites of potential infection in the diabetic presenting with DKA, especially chest, feet (remove shoes and socks), perianal region and urine (dipstick for nitrites).

> Abdominal – is there abdominal tenderness, silent bowel sounds or pain in the renal angles? Has an intra-abdominal event triggered the

DKA? In addition to infection/ peritonitis, do not forget bowel infarction – particularly if there is a background of diabetic macrovascular disease. Do not forget a rectal examination: you will not see a perianal abscess unless you look.

Key point

Remember that DKA can mimic an acute abdomen.

> Neurological – check the GCS score to assess this. Also check for the presence of meningeal irritation or focal signs, which would be unlikely but of great significance if present.

There may be signs of chronic damage caused by diabetes – eg retinopathy, neuropathy or vascular disease – but examining for these is not a high priority in the context of the patient presenting with DKA.

Investigations

Key point

Diabetic ketoacidosis (DKA) is diagnosed by the presence of hyperglycaemia (glucose >11 mmol/L), acidosis (bicarbonate <15 mmol/L or pH <7.30) and ketonaemia (ketones >3.0 mmol/L).

Urinary and capillary blood ketones

Significant ketonuria, detected by finding 2+ or greater result on Ketostix testing, supports the diagnosis of DKA. Best practice is to test capillary ketones with point-of-care devices: >3 mmol/L ketones is in keeping with a diagnosis of DKA.

Routine blood tests

Blood glucose (laboratory) – often the finger-prick blood glucose will read high without a precise value.

Electrolytes and renal function – the serum potassium is likely to be high at presentation, but remember that the total body potassium will be significantly depleted; expect the urea to be elevated out of proportion to the creatinine because of dehydration; and compare the creatinine with any previous measurements to determine if renal impairment is acute, chronic or acute on chronic.

Full blood count (FBC) – a raised white cell count might suggest sepsis but can be elevated in the absence of infection in DKA.

Other – CRP to confirm suspicion of sepsis. Liver/bone profiles.

Sepsis screen

Send urine for microscopy and culture, blood cultures and other cultures as appropriate, eg sputum and wound swabs.

Chest radiograph, looking for evidence of infection and also for air under the diaphragm: perforation of an abdominal viscus can be remarkably silent in a diabetic.

Venous blood gases

DKA produces a metabolic acidosis with respiratory compensation. The presence of ketone bodies results in a high anion gap, calculated as $(Na^+ + K^+) - (Cl^- + HCO_3^-)$, with normal range 10–8 mmol/L. In most cases of DKA, ABGs are not necessary.

Other investigations

Although it is likely to be normal in this young woman, check an ECG: MI can be a precipitant of DKA and electrolyte disorders can result in arrhythmias. Also perform other imaging tests, eg urinary tract ultrasonography and bone radiographs, as dictated by clinical suspicion.

Management

Key point

Priorities of management in a patient with DKA:

> ABC

> correction of hypovolaemia with intravenous fluids

> correction of hyperglycaemia with a fixed-rate insulin infusion

> continuation of long-acting insulin analogues as normal

> meticulous correction of electrolyte imbalance, particularly potassium

> treatment of any underlying cause

> prophylaxis against venous thromboembolism

> involvement of the diabetes specialist team as early as possible.

Fluid resuscitation and electrolyte replacement, particularly potassium

Patients with DKA are severely dehydrated and very deplete of total body sodium and potassium: fluid replacement is the top priority. Proceed as described in Section 1.3.13 if hypovolaemic shock is present, but most patients are not profoundly hypotensive and should be given 0.9% saline (normal saline) with additional potassium in most cases. Typical requirements in the first 24 hours are as shown in Table 13, but the patient will require frequent clinical reassessment over this time and the fluid regimen may need to be adjusted.

Table 13	Fluid replacement in diabetic ketoacidosis		
Fluid	**Volume**	**Time**	**Potassium replacement**
0.9% saline	1 L	1 hour	None with first litre, then potassium (K) as determined by serum K⁺ measurement as follows:
0.9% saline	1 L	2 hour	
0.9% saline	1 L	4 hour	
0.9% saline	1 L	4 hour	
0.9% saline	1 L	4 hour	
0.9% saline	1 L	4 hour	
0.9% saline	1 L	4 hour	

Serum K^+ (mmol/L)	K^+ added (mmol to each L)
<3.5	40
3.5–5.0	20
>5	None

Key point

DKA leads to a negative potassium balance through osmotic diuresis and acidaemia. There will be a rapid decline in serum potassium concentration as it re-enters cells in the first few hours of treatment with rehydration and insulin. Potassium must be replaced as part of the fluid regimen, guided by frequent monitoring of serum potassium throughout treatment.

Correction of hyperglycaemia

Insulin therapy reverses ketogenesis, lowers the blood sugar and stops osmotic diuresis. Commence a fixed-rate insulin infusion (Table 14) and monitoring of blood sugar hourly by the finger-prick method. Note that the insulin infusion should be continued until the serum and urine are clear of ketones and metabolic acidosis has been corrected: this may mean persisting with it after normoglycaemia has been achieved, which can be done if intravenous dextrose replaces 0.9% saline as indicated in Table 13.

Correction of acid–base disturbance

Insulin reverses ketogenesis and causes oxidation of existing ketones, resulting in endogenous bicarbonate production. Restoration of normovolaemia will rapidly reverse the lactate component of metabolic acidosis if there is adequate renal function and tissue perfusion. Treatment with alkali is not routinely required.

Hazard

Bicarbonate administration should not be routinely used in DKA – it may cause exacerbation of hypokalaemia, paradoxical intracellular acidosis due to increased carbon dioxide production, shift of the oxygen dissociation curve to the left and late alkalosis.

Table 14	Insulin infusion for the treatment of diabetic ketoacidosis
Patient weight (kg)	**Insulin dose (U/h)**
60–69	6
70–79	7
80–89	8
90–99	9
100–109	10
110–119	11
120–129	12
130–139	13
140–150	14
>150	15

Dilute 50 units of soluble insulin (Actrapid) in 50 mL normal saline and give at the rate indicated (which may need to be adjusted depending on the patient's response).

Treat infection

Infection is a common precipitant of DKA, particularly pneumonia, urinary tract infection (including pyelonephritis and perinephric abscess), skin sepsis and abscesses. Remember that patients with diabetes may not manifest the classical signs of infection. Have a low threshold for starting empirical broad-spectrum antibiotics after a full septic screen.

Prophylaxis against thromboembolism

An immobile dehydrated patient is at high risk of venous thromboembolism: start low-molecular-weight heparin (prophylactic dose).

Consider risk of aspiration

Diabetic patients with autonomic neuropathy are at high risk of having an atonic stomach, which can contain a large volume of acidic content that can be fatal if aspirated. If the patient is nauseous or vomiting, then consider inserting a nasogastric (NG) tube to empty the stomach.

Further comments

Cerebral oedema

This is a rare but feared complication of DKA, mostly reported in children or young adults and with a high mortality. Suspect it if the patent complains of a headache or becomes increasingly drowsy and confused. Excessive rehydration and hypertonic fluids can sometimes be responsible. ICU advice and transfer should be requested urgently if cerebral oedema is suspected.

Hyperosmolar hyperglycaemic state

Hyperosmolar hyperglycaemic state (HHS) must be considered in any case of severe hyperglycaemia. It is typically seen in older patients with non-insulin-dependent diabetes and is commonly precipitated by intercurrent illness. Various medications (eg thiazide diuretics and steroids) and consumption of glucose-rich fluids, eg Lucozade, can also precipitate it. Patients are not (by definition) ketoacidotic, but may be acidotic due to lactate accumulation as a result of poor tissue perfusion. The approach to investigation and management is similar to that for DKA, but there are additional points to bear in mind.

Diagnosis

Plasma osmolality, calculated as $2 \times (Na^+ + K^+) + glucose + urea$, is >320 mOsm/kg. Glucose is >30 mmol/L. There may be marked hypernatraemia. Dehydration tends to be severe, causing a disproportionately raised plasma urea. Arterial blood gases (ABGs) are usually relatively normal with pH >7.3 and HCO_3^- >15 mmol/L unless there is significant lactate accumulation. Unlike DKA, ketonaemia is modest or absent (<3 mmol/L).

Treatment

The use of hypotonic fluid for rehydration is controversial, the fear being that over-rapid reduction of hypernatraemia may result in neurological damage or death. The safest approach is to use 0.9% (normal) saline initially to restore BP and urine flow, and then to change to 0.45% saline if plasma sodium is still >150 mmol/L. Insulin requirements may be low, hence start at a lower dose of insulin and monitor the finger-prick blood glucose closely to avoid hypoglycaemia. Patients with HHS are particularly prone to thromboembolism: anticoagulate with low-molecular-weight heparin as routine.

Why did it happen?

Key point

Diabetic patients do not develop DKA or HHS overnight: it builds up over several days. In those known to have diabetes, these dangerous conditions are almost invariably avoidable and when a patient has recovered from an episode they should not leave hospital without advice about how to avoid another.

Key point

Advice to diabetics to prevent DKA or HHS:

> If you get ill, you are likely to need more insulin rather than less.

> If you get ill, check your blood sugar at least four times a day.

> If the blood sugar is going up and you do not know what to do – call for help.

1.3.19 Hypoglycaemia

Case history

A 70-year-old woman with non-insulin-dependent diabetes is brought to the emergency department after being found unconscious on the kitchen floor. During transfer to hospital she had a generalised seizure and on arrival she is unresponsive to pain.

Introduction

Key point

After checking airway, breathing and circulation (ABC), and then considering opioid toxicity (pinpoint pupils and low respiratory rate) and drug overdose, checking a finger-prick blood glucose to diagnose or exclude hypoglycaemia is the next priority in dealing with the unconscious patient (Fig 32).

The general approach to the unconscious patient is described in Section 1.3.29. This clinical scenario deals with those issues specific to the patient with hypoglycaemia.

History of the presenting problem

Key point

Treat hypoglycaemia first…ask questions afterwards.

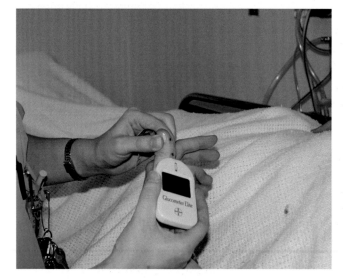

Fig 32 Do not ever forget to check a finger-prick blood glucose in a patient who is unconscious.

A patient in hypoglycaemic coma will not be able to give a history! After immediate treatment they may be able to give an account of themselves, but still may not remember key details. Hence ensure that anyone who might know what happened does not disappear from the department while you are treating the patient. Important aspects to ask about are:

> History of diabetes – is the patient prone to hypoglycaemia?

> Treatment for diabetes – has this been changed recently?

> Possible precipitating cause, eg alcohol intake or concurrent illness.

> Could they have taken an overdose of their medication, either accidental or deliberate?

Examination

As described in Section 1.3.29. Once the patient has responded to treatment, perform a full neurological examination: neurological deficit may persist for days or weeks, and is sometimes permanent, despite correction of the blood sugar in cases of severe, prolonged hypoglycaemia.

Investigations

Hypoglycaemia most commonly arises in known diabetics, who respond rapidly to treatment. Such cases typically require no investigation beyond confirming hypoglycaemia with a finger-prick blood test. By contrast, the hypoglycaemic diabetic who does not respond to glucose requires consideration of other diagnoses, as described in Section 1.3.29.

A much rarer scenario is the patient with hypoglycaemia demonstrated on a finger-prick blood test who is not known to be a diabetic. In such cases, the differential diagnoses listed in Table 15 should be considered, and blood should be drawn for the following tests before dextrose is given if at all possible (but do not delay treatment while you wait for the results):

> laboratory blood glucose

> serum to be saved for insulin and C-peptide levels.

Management

Key point

Urgent treatment is vital if permanent cerebral damage is to be avoided – any patient with a finger-prick blood glucose reading of <2.5 mmol/L who is unconscious should be given 100 mL 20% dextrose or 200 mL 10% dextrose over 10–15 minutes. 50% dextrose is no longer recommended (but 50 mL 50% dextrose should be given if readily available and 10 or 20% preparations are not). In some centres, 1 mg IM glucagon can be given in an emergency for those without intravenous access, but note this takes 15 minutes to take effect and will not work if the hypoglycaemia is due to alcohol.

For patients with hypoglycaemia who are conscious and able to swallow, options include fruit juice, Dextrogel or GlucoGel.

Hazard

A patient who is unconscious with a blood glucose reading of >1.5 mmol/L is unlikely to be unconscious due to hypoglycaemia – but you cannot be 100% sure, and there can be a terrible penalty for not treating hypoglycaemic coma. If in doubt, treat!

Hazard

Hypoglycaemia in the 'down and out' – if there is a history of chronic high alcohol intake or malnourishment, give thiamine intravenously before glucose to avoid precipitating Wernicke's encephalopathy.

Note that the half-lives of oral hypoglycaemic agents, and medium- and long-acting insulin preparations are both longer than that of glucose. The patient should not be discharged the moment that they become conscious: give them a sugary drink and something to eat to prevent recurrent hypoglycaemia, and monitor them for at least a few hours (how long will depend on the reason for hypoglycaemia and the social circumstances to which the patient would be discharged). Recheck their glucose 15–30 minutes after treatment and start an infusion of 10% dextrose – aiming to maintain blood glucose at 5–10 mmol/L – if hypoglycaemia recurs.

Further comments

Why did it happen?

Hypoglycaemia can strike diabetics out of the blue, but most have some warning. Before the patient is discharged, talk through with them what (if anything) they remember about the event. Impress on them that hypoglycaemia is serious – it can be fatal. Tell them that if they get the same feelings again they must check their blood sugar, and that they must have some sugar available to take at all times. With the patient's permission, it is also prudent to offer advice and instruction on how to recognise and handle hypoglycaemia to any of their close family and friends.

1.3.20 Hypercalcaemia

Case history

A 58-year-old man is taken to see his GP by his daughter because he has become increasingly confused and lethargic over the past 5 days. Blood tests are checked, following which the biochemistry department phones the doctor on call for the practice to say that the serum corrected calcium is 3.8 mmol/L (normal range 2.20–2.60 mmol/L). The patient is sent immediately to the emergency department where you are asked to review him.

Introduction

Consider the causes of hypercalcaemia – particularly the common ones – as you take the history, examine and investigate (Table 16).

Table 15 Causes of hypoglycaemia

Diabetic patients	Non-diabetic patients
Insulin Oral hypoglycaemics (especially longer-acting sulfonylureas) Sudden withdrawal of steroids Excessive alcohol intake Excessive exercise Specific inpatient causes include lack of bedtime snacks, being given regular insulin doses (which have been avoided at home) and being made 'nil by mouth' prior to surgery	Concealed insulin administration Drugs (eg oral hypoglycaemics, quinine and pentamidine) Salicylate overdose Excessive alcohol (especially chronic alcoholics with liver disease) Sepsis Insulinoma Retroperitoneal sarcoma Hypopituitarism Adrenocortical insufficiency Hypothyroidism Liver failure Eating disorders such as anorexia nervosa

Table 16 Causes of hypercalcaemia

Cause	Condition
Common	Hyperparathyroidism – primary or tertiary Malignancy – primary or secondary, and especially myeloma, lung and breast Sarcoidosis
Less common/rare	Other granulomatous diseases Excess vitamin D Drugs – particularly thiazide diuretics and lithium Milk/alkali syndrome Other endocrine disorders – thyrotoxicosis, phaeochromocytoma and acute adrenal insufficiency Immobilisation Inappropriate PTH levels due to altered set point – familial benign hypocalciuric hypercalcaemia

PTH, parathyroid hormone.

History of the presenting problem

The patient will probably only be able to give a limited history, but ask him and his daughter about symptoms caused by hypercalcaemia. Acute hypercalcaemia can cause fatigue, apathy, anorexia, thirst, polyuria and constipation; with nausea, vomiting, confusion and coma in severe cases. Symptoms of chronic hypercalcaemia include abdominal pain, urinary stones and depression.

Other relevant history

Are there any clues as to the cause of the hypercalcaemia? Consider the diagnoses listed in Table 16 as you enquire about:

> Previous history of malignancy.

> Symptoms of malignancy, eg weight loss, back/bone pain, chest or abdominal symptoms – these are usually present when hypercalcaemia is due to cancer.

> Speed of onset of problems – a short history is more typical of hypercalcaemia of malignancy than hypercalcaemia associated with hyperparathyroidism and other diseases.

> Drugs – is the patient receiving thiazide diuretics, vitamin D or lithium?

> Other medications – does the patient have a history of indigestion, and if so are they treating it with over-the-counter remedies or 'white medicine'?

> Is there a concurrent disease predisposing to dehydration or immobility?

Key point

A thorough drug history is essential – patients often do not regard over-the-counter remedies as drugs, particularly ones for a problem as common as indigestion.

Although it seems very likely that this man's confusion is related to his hypercalcaemia, do not forget to consider other possibilities, eg sepsis (could he have pneumonia or a urinary tract infection?), drug side effects (is he on opioids or anything else that might cause confusion?) and other effects of malignancy (eg headache may indicate cerebral metastases).

Examination

Begin with an overall assessment, as described in Section 1.3.2, but key issues will be to assess fluid status, where volume depletion is likely, and to look for evidence of malignancy:

Fluid status

> Intravascular volume – check pulse, BP (lying and sitting/standing) and JVP.

> Interstitial/intracellular fluid volume – check skin turgor and mucous membranes.

Evidence of malignancy

The symptoms will point to the type of malignancy:

> general – cachexia, lymphadenopathy and hepatomegaly

> lung cancer – clubbing, Horner's syndrome and chest signs

> breast examination.

Clues to other specific causes of confusion and drowsiness

Check pupils and respiratory rate – small pupils and a low respiratory rate probably mean opioid toxicity. If these features are present, give naloxone as described in Section 1.3.29. Look carefully at the fundi – papilloedema suggests raised intracranial pressure. Any clear focal neurological signs would suggest cerebral metastasis in this clinical context.

Investigations

Repeat the measurement of serum calcium to confirm hypercalcaemia; also check electrolytes and renal function (acute renal failure is commonly seen in severe hypercalcaemia), liver/bone profile, FBC (anaemia may be present for several reasons, most commonly malignant involvement of bone marrow), inflammatory markers, parathyroid hormone (PTH) and serum immunoglobulins/serum protein electrophoresis/urinary Bence Jones proteins. Perform a chest radiograph, looking in particular for evidence of malignancy (Fig 33) or features of sarcoidosis.

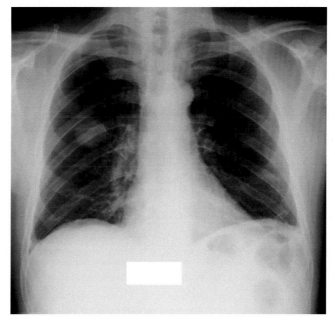

Fig 33 Chest radiograph showing bronchogenic carcinoma.

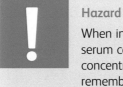

Hazard

When interpreting serum calcium concentration, remember:

> Free (ionised) plasma calcium is dependent on plasma albumin.

> Corrected calcium = measured calcium + ([40 – serum albumin (g/L)] × 0.02).

In most cases the cause of hypercalcaemia will be established by the history, examination and the investigations listed above, but in selected cases the following further tests may be needed: 25-hydroxyvitamin D3, thyroid function tests, PTH-related peptide serum ACE, serum magnesium, urinary calcium and creatinine excretion, and bone radiographs.

In any sick patient an ECG should also be performed. In severe hypercalcaemia this can show slowed conduction, including prolonged P-R interval, and a widened QRS complex and shortened Q-T interval with ST-segments shortened or absent. Bradyarrhythmias, bundle branch block and atrioventricular (AV) block may develop as the serum calcium rises to around 4.50 mmol/L.

Other tests, eg sepsis screen, ABGs and CT brain scan, may be required depending on clinical suspicion.

Management

Key point

Principles of emergency management of hypercalcaemia

> Increase urinary excretion of calcium by rehydration with 0.9% saline.

> Inhibit bone resorption with bisphosphonate therapy.

Urgent treatment of hypercalcaemia is needed if there is a reduced consciousness level, confusion, intravascular volume depletion or gross dehydration, or if the patient's serum calcium is >3.5 mmol/L (most patients will be symptomatic at this stage).

Rehydration

The first aspect of emergency management should be rehydration with intravenous saline as follows:

> Correct intravascular volume depletion – if this is present (postural tachycardia/hypotension and low JVP) give 0.9% (normal) saline rapidly until the patient is replete (see Section 1.3.2).

> When intravascular volume depletion is corrected – give 0.9% (normal) saline IV at a rate of around 3–6 L in 24 hours if the patient has a satisfactory urine output. Insert a urinary catheter to monitor urine output. Consider giving furosemide 40–80 mg IV to encourage diuresis. Examine the patient regularly for signs of fluid overload or deficit, ensure accurate fluid charts are kept and adjust fluid input accordingly.

> Monitor the calcium level and also the levels of potassium and magnesium, which may fall rapidly with rehydration. Replace as necessary.

Bisphosphonate therapy

Bisphosphonates are one of the most effective drugs for controlling hypercalcaemia: they bind to hydroxyapatite in calcified bone, which renders it resistant to dissolution thereby inhibiting both normal and abnormal bone resorption. They have a slow onset of action (1–3 days) but can have a prolonged effect (12–30 days). Disodium pamidronate is the first-choice drug for hypercalcaemia associated with malignancy: 30–90 mg IV is given slowly (over 2–6 hours with 0.5 L 0.9% saline) into a large vein.

Calcitonin

Calcitonin can be useful in the short-term management of the patient with severe hypercalcaemia: it rapidly (in 2–4 hours) inhibits calcium and phosphorous resorption from the bone and decreases renal calcium reabsorption. The initial dose schedule is 4 IU/kg of body weight per dose, which is administered subcutaneously or intramuscularly every 12 hours. The dose and schedule may be escalated after 1 or 2 days to 8 IU/kg every 12 hours, and finally to 8 IU/kg every 6 hours if the response to lower doses is unsatisfactory. Unfortunately, tachyphylaxis commonly occurs and reduced hypocalcaemic effect is seen with further dosing, meaning that the calcium-lowering effects of calcitonin last for only a few days.

Glucocorticoids

Glucocorticoids are the treatment of choice for hypercalcaemia caused by vitamin D toxicity, sarcoidosis or myeloma. Give hydrocortisone 200 mg IV or prednisolone 40–60 mg orally.

Key point

Effect of steroids on hypercalcaemia
The main mechanism of action of steroids is to decrease 1,25-dihydroxyvitamin-D levels by inhibiting inflammatory cell proliferation within granulomatous tissue and haematological malignancies. Although the steroids also decrease intestinal calcium absorption and increase urinary calcium excretion, this occurs relatively slowly.

1.3.21 Hyponatraemia

Case history

A 70-year-old man is brought into the emergency department after being found unconscious on a park bench. He has a history of alcohol abuse and is known to have attended the emergency department following a minor head injury 4 weeks previously. He is confused, but is moving all his limbs and trying to get off the trolley. He smells strongly of alcohol. No obvious head injury is apparent and he has no focal neurological signs.

His finger-prick blood glucose is 6.9 mmol/L. He has routine bloods taken and is sent to the clinical decision unit pending results and his progress. The nursing staff bleep you with his electrolyte results – sodium 110 mmol/L (normal range 137–144), potassium 3.2 mmol/L (normal range 3.5–4.9) and urea 2.0 mmol/L (normal range 2.5–7.0).

Introduction

The general approach to the unconscious patient is described in Section 1.3.29. This clinical scenario deals with those issues specific to the patient with hyponatraemia.

Patients vary in their susceptibility to hyponatraemia. Gradual, chronic lowering of the serum sodium concentration is generally much better tolerated than a rapid, acute fall; hence symptoms depend not simply on the sodium concentration but its rate of change. However, patients with mild hyponatraemia (sodium 125–135 mmol/L) are usually asymptomatic; those with moderate hyponatraemia (sodium 115–125 mmol/L) may have nausea, malaise, headache, lethargy, restlessness and disorientation; and those with severe hyponatraemia (sodium <115 mmol/L) may suffer seizure, coma and death.

Key point

The critical things to know about hyponatraemia are:

> Patients with hyponatraemia have too much water on board – they are almost never short of sodium.

> Hyponatraemia that has developed slowly is often well tolerated and, if this is the case, should be corrected slowly, usually with water restriction alone.

> Hyponatraemia that has developed quickly is relatively rare, often iatrogenic and is much more likely to cause symptoms. If it is symptomatic then rapid correction with hypertonic saline is likely to be required, with care to avoid overcorrection. This is because patients with chronic hyponatraemia that has been overcorrected are most at risk of dire neurological consequences.

Consider the causes of hyponatraemia (Tables 17 and 18) as you try to work out the cause of the problem.

Hazard

Cause of severe acute hyponatraemia
The commonest cause is iatrogenic–postoperative infusion of excessive volumes of 5% dextrose solution. Non-osmotic stimuli for ADH release include haemorrhage, nausea, pain and anaesthesia, all of which can be present immediately after operations, leading to enormously high levels of ADH and an inability to excrete water. If a doctor then prescribes large volumes of 5% dextrose the consequences can be dire.

History and examination

This man will clearly not be able to give a reliable history. Proceed with history and examination as described in Section 1.3.29, but – referring to Tables 17 and 18 – important issues to consider particularly in this case are: could he have a subdural haematoma?; could he have been vomiting (is there evidence of intravascular volume depletion)?; does he have cirrhosis/liver failure or renal failure (what do the notes from his last attendance reveal)?; and has he been on treatment with diuretics?

Investigation

This man's neurological state may simply reflect the fact that he is drunk, but it would be unwise to assume that this is the explanation given his profound hyponatraemia. The standard approach to investigation of the unconscious patient is described in Section 1.3.29, but in this case consider the following.

CT brain scan
It would be appropriate to image the brain even in the absence of focal neurological signs given that this man is an alcoholic with a history of recent head injury and that subdural haematoma can be associated with syndrome of inappropriate antidiuretic hormone (SIADH).

Cause of hyponatraemia
Urinary sodium concentration (urine 'spot sodium') is useful to distinguish between renal and extrarenal hypovolaemic hyponatraemia, as well as between causes of hypervolaemic hyponatraemia (see Table 17). Paired urine and plasma osmolarities should be sent along with the spot sodium: measurement of these is required to pursue the possibility of SIADH (it is important to remember that this is a diagnosis of exclusion – see below). Further investigations will depend on underlying suspected cause.

Key point

The criteria for the diagnosis of SIADH – all must be satisfied to confirm the diagnosis:

> Plasma osmolality is <270 mOsm/kg with inappropriate urinary concentration (>100 mOsm/kg).

> Patient is euvolaemic and not taking a diuretic.

> Renal sodium excretion is >20 mmol/L.

> Normal renal, thyroid and adrenal function.

Table 17 Causes of hyponatraemia

Volume status	Total body water	Total extracellular sodium	Primary problem	Example
Hypovolaemic	Low	Even lower	Renal – urinary Na >30 mmol/L	Diuretics
				Sodium-losing renal disorders
				Mineralocorticoid deficiency
			Non-renal – urinary Na <30 mmol/L	Vomiting
				Diarrhoea
				Burns
				Excessive sweating
Euvolaemic	Normal/slight excess	Reduced/normal		SIADH
				Glucocorticoid deficiency
				Hypothyroidism
				'Sick cells'
Hypervolaemic	Great excess	Excess	Renal – urinary Na >30 mmol/L	Acute/chronic renal failure
			Non-renal – urinary Na <30 mmol/L	Cardiac failure
				Cirrhosis/liver failure
				Nephrotic syndrome

Note that in all cases the development of hyponatraemia requires fluid replacement with hypotonic fluid (by drinking of water or 5% dextrose infusion)
SIADH, syndrome of inappropriate antidiuretic hormone.

Table 18 Causes of SIADH

Source of ADH	Type of problem	Example
Ectopic ADH production	Malignancy	Small-cell lung cancer
Inappropriate pituitary ADH secretion	Malignancy	Lung cancer, lymphoma, prostate cancer and pancreatic cancer
	Inflammatory lung disease	Pneumonia and lung abscess
	Neurological disease	Meningitis, head injury, subdural haematoma, tumours and post-surgery
	Drugs	Antidepressants (tricyclics and SSRIs), carbamazepine, chlorpropamide, phenothiazines (eg chlorpromazine), vincristine, cyclophosphamide and ecstasy
	Postoperative[1]	–
	Others	Nausea, pain and porphyria

1 See the 'Cause of severe acute hyponatraemia' hazard box above.
ADH, antidiuretic hormone; SIADH, syndrome of inappropriate antidiuretic hormone; SSRIs, selective serotonin reuptake inhibitors.

Management

The correct strategy for management of hyponatraemia depends on whether or not the patient is symptomatic as a result of it. Harm can be done by overzealous correction: in the case of an older woman who is relatively well but hyponatraemic due to diuretic treatment, she is much more likely to suffer than to benefit from an aggressive medical approach. This is a difficult case: he is probably symptomatic as a result of severe acute hyponatraemia and should be treated as such, while remaining alert to the fact that there could be other reasons for his mental state.

Asymptomatic hyponatraemia

Management of the patient with asymptomatic hyponatraemia depends on identifying and treating (where possible) the underlying cause (Table 17), coupled with restriction of fluid input to 1 L/day to enable the serum sodium concentration to rise. Such fluid restriction can be difficult for patients to tolerate and for nurses to enforce: give the allocation in aliquots throughout the day; give it as ice cubes to suck; and permit the patient swabs to keep their mouth moist or to suck boiled sweets.

Key point

Hyponatraemia alone is very unlikely to cause neurological symptoms unless the concentration is <120 mmol/L – if the serum sodium concentration is higher than this in a comatose patient, consider other causes of coma.

Symptomatic hyponatraemia

Urgent treatment is required if there are severe neurological effects, eg fitting. Aside from treating the underlying cause, use hypertonic saline to bring up the patient's serum sodium concentration. However, remember that central pontine myelinolysis is reported in association with overrapid correction and note the following:

> No formula can accurately predict the patient's response to being given hypertonic saline – all of them assume a 'closed system' and take no account of the patient's ongoing water losses, which are not predictable.

> 1.8% saline infused at a rate of 1.7 mL/kg/h or 3% saline infused at a rate of 1 mL/kg/h is likely to increase the serum sodium concentration by 1 mmol/L/h.

> Aim to bring the serum sodium concentration up in the early stages of correction by about 1 mmol/L/h and by no more than 8–10 mmol/L over 24 hours.

> Monitor the serum sodium concentration every 2 hours while infusing hypertonic saline, and replace the hypertonic saline with 0.9% saline if the serum sodium is rising more quickly than desired.

> Stop the infusion of hypertonic saline when the serum sodium is >125 mmol/L and institute water restriction: do not allow rapid correction into the normal range.

Hazard

Treatment of severe hyponatraemia
Correction of symptomatic hyponatraemia with hypertonic saline requires very close monitoring – check serum sodium every 2 hours.

1.3.22 Addisonian crisis

Case history

A 32-year-old woman is brought to the emergency department by her husband. He explains that she collapsed today at work and was sent home. She has been unwell for some time with lethargy and dizziness, and she has lost a significant amount of weight. On arrival she is drowsy, confused and complaining of abdominal pain. She looks unwell and has BP 80/50 mmHg. Urgent bloods are taken by the physician's assistant. You are in the process of assessing her when the biochemistry results become available, showing sodium 128 mmol/L (normal range 137–144) and potassium 5.8 mmol/L (normal range 3.5–4.9).

Introduction

The clinical approach to the patient with hypotension is discussed in Section 1.3.2, but in this case there are a number of clues that this is an 'acute on chronic' presentation: the patient has been unwell for some time suggesting a chronic disease process, and there are clear clues to acute adrenal insufficiency (Addisonian crisis) – hypotension with mild hyponatraemia and hyperkalaemia.

History of presenting complaint

A thorough history is obviously required, but the information available means that you should enquire carefully about features that would support the diagnosis of adrenal insufficiency.

Features suggesting chronic adrenal insufficiency

Non-specific symptoms are a dominant feature: dizziness on standing caused by postural hypotension is common; many patients report constipation or diarrhoea; and progressive weight loss can be an important clue to the insidious development of the disease. If asked directly many patients will report a craving for salt.

Features suggesting Addisonian crisis

About 25% of patients with Addison's disease present in crisis, with rapid progression of their symptoms. Many cases develop non-specific abdominal pain in conjunction with nausea and/or vomiting; and also restlessness and confusion, which in some patients can progress to stupor and coma.

Is there any history to suggest an underlying precipitant to the crisis?

Any intercurrent illness may precipitate an Addisonian crisis, when in rare cases a history of flank pain may be due to haemorrhagic adrenal infarction.

Other relevant history

Drug history

Previous steroid usage may have caused adrenal suppression and left the patient vulnerable to an Addisonian crisis in the event of intercurrent illness. Rifampicin and ketoconazole can also cause primary hypoadrenalism in some patients.

Key point

Patients on long-term steroids require additional steroids to cover intercurrent illness/stress.

Autoimmune diseases

In the UK autoimmune disease accounts for about 80% of cases of Addison's disease, in which it is associated with other autoimmune conditions including vitiligo, pernicious anaemia, thyroiditis, type 1 diabetes mellitus and hypoparathyroidism.

Other possible underlying causes

Tuberculosis (TB) and malignancy can cause adrenal failure.

Examination

Resuscitation as described in Section 1.3.2 will be the immediate priority, but in view of the suspicion of Addison's disease in this case you should, aside from concentrating on the state of the circulation and looking for evidence of sepsis as a precipitant of crisis, look carefully for pigmentation (Fig 34) and also for vitiligo.

Given the presentation with abdominal pain it will clearly be important to check carefully for signs of intra-abdominal mischief.

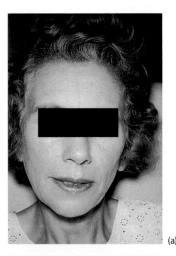

(a)

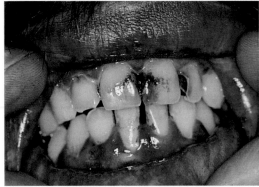

(c)

Investigation

The approach to investigation of the very ill patient is described in Section 1.3.2, but in this case particularly consider the following.

Routine investigation of the ill patient

Blood glucose may be low, with symptomatic hypoglycaemia. Electrolytes / renal function tests classically show hyponatraemia, hyperkalaemia (as in this case) and a high urea, but they can be normal. Hypercalcaemia can be seen in conjunction with significant dehydration, but is sometimes seen after rehydration. FBC may show anaemia, or a raised white cell count if there is an infective precipitant. The chest radiograph is likely to show a small heart and may show pneumonia as a precipitant of crisis. Adrenal calcification from old TB may be visible on an abdominal radiograph.

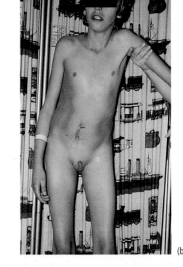

(b)

Fig 34 Hyperpigmentation of the skin (a, b) and buccal tissues (c) in patients with Addison's disease.

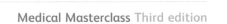

Key point

The typical findings in acute adrenal insufficiency are hyponatraemia, hyperkalaemia and hypoglycaemia.

Establishing the diagnosis of adrenal insufficiency

> Random cortisol measurement – if possible take a sample before administration of steroid, but remember that random cortisol measurements are difficult to interpret and should be viewed with caution.

> Short adrenocorticotropic hormone (ACTH; Synacthen) stimulation test – in this case it would be dangerous and wrong to delay treatment, but in less dramatic circumstances this should be done as a priority if adrenal insufficiency is suspected. Synacthen (0.25 mg) is administered IM/IV to the patient (time 0); samples for measurement of plasma cortisol are collected at 0, +30 and +60 minutes; a cortisol level >550 nmol/L (with rise from baseline >190 nmol/L) excludes the diagnosis of primary adrenal failure.

> Plasma ACTH – a high level (>80 ng/L) with low or low-normal cortisol confirms primary hypoadrenalism.

It will be appropriate to check thyroid function in all cases of adrenal insufficiency. If hydrocortisone is given acutely, as should be done in this case, then short (or long) Synacthen testing can be done at a later date after the omission of hydrocortisone for 24 hours or substitution with dexamethasone. Further endocrinological investigations, eg pituitary function tests, will be required in selected cases.

Management

Key aspects of resuscitation in this case are:

> Fluids – the patient in Addisonian crisis is significantly depleted of both salt and water: aggressive fluid resuscitation with 0.9% saline is vital.

> Glucocorticoid replacement – give hydrocortisone 100–200 mg IV immediately, and then 100 mg IV three times daily. Fludrocortisone replacement will need to be considered in the long term, but in the acute situation hydrocortisone is the treatment of choice.

> Beware of the risk of hypoglycaemia – monitor the finger-prick blood glucose regularly; put up a 10% dextrose drip if necessary and run it at a rate to keep the glucose >5 mmol/L, but do not give more than is needed and avoid using 5% dextrose because it is more likely to exacerbate hyponatraemia.

> Consider sepsis – have a low threshold for treating with empirical antibiotics.

Hazard

Shoot first – ask questions afterwards Give steroids immediately if you suspect Addisonian crisis.

1.3.23 Thyrotoxic crisis

Case history

A 45-year-old woman is brought to the emergency department because she has become increasingly paranoid over the past few days. She is known to have 'a thyroid problem' but has recently become interested in homeopathic medicine and stopped taking her usual tablets. She is agitated and delusional, so taking a history is not straightforward, but she has clearly lost a lot of weight, has a marked tremor, is febrile and is tachycardic. You are asked to assess her urgently by the nurse in charge.

History of the presenting problem

Getting a detailed history is not possible in this case, but the problem is clear cut: features of a thyrotoxic crisis (storm) include weight loss, heat intolerance, sweating, palpitations, diarrhoea, tremor and anxiety/agitation/irritability.

Possible precipitating causes of a thyrotoxic crisis include withdrawal of antithyroid drug therapy (as in this case), but also infection, radioiodine treatment, iodinated contrast dyes, thyroid surgery and childbirth.

Examination

The approach to the examination of the very ill patient is described in Section 1.3.2, but in this case you would obviously look for features that would be consistent with a diagnosis of thyrotoxic crisis:

> General – agitation, anxiety and restlessness; tremor; the skin is usually warm and moist; and hyperpyrexia – a feature of thyrotoxic crisis and does not necessarily indicate infection, although this should always be looked for.

> Cardiovascular compromise – sinus tachycardia is usually greater than 140 beats per minute in thyroid crisis (storm); fast atrial fibrillation (AF) or supraventricular tachycardia (SVT) are common; is there cardiac failure – raised JVP, gallop rhythm, pulmonary oedema and peripheral oedema?

> Neurological/psychological – altered consciousness, frank psychosis, delirium, seizures and coma can all be seen in thyrotoxic crisis.

Findings that might indicate the likely cause of the thyroid pathology are:

> Signs of Graves' disease (Fig 35) – exophthalmos, eyelid retraction and lid lag.

> Is there a goitre? If so, what are its characteristics (smooth, nodular or painful), and is there an associated bruit?

> Vitiligo – associated with autoimmune thyroid disease.

Investigation

Hazard

Thyrotoxic crisis is a clinical diagnosis
There are no laboratory criteria to diagnose thyrotoxic crisis – the levels of thyroid hormones are the same as in uncomplicated hyperthyroidism. Start treatment immediately if the clinical diagnosis is thyrotoxic crisis: do not delay while waiting for laboratory confirmation.

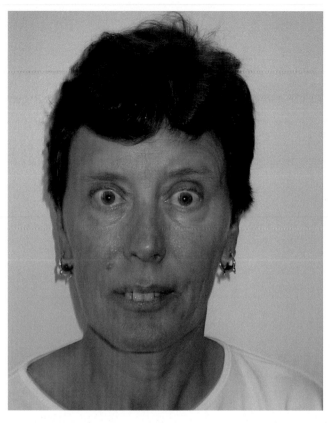

Fig 35 A patient with exophthalmos and lid retraction due to Graves' disease.

The approach to investigation of the very ill patient is described in Section 1.3.2, but in this case the following would be particularly important:

> ECG – sinus tachycardia is expected, but look for AF or other arrhythmia.

> Thyroid function tests – clear evidence of hyperthyroidism would be expected, but in this clinical context you should not wait for confirmation before beginning treatment.

Management

Thyrotoxic crisis is a life-threatening condition, with mortality of up to 20–30% reported. Aside from basic resuscitation (see Section 1.3.2), give specific treatment for thyrotoxic crisis on clinical suspicion.

Hyperthyroidism
The patient in thyrotoxic crisis requires both of the following:

> Propylthiouracil or carbimazole – propylthiouracil is the preferred drug as it both blocks further synthesis of thyroid hormones and inhibits peripheral T4 to T3 conversion. However, it is often not immediately available on the wards, whereas carbimazole usually is. If propylthiouracil is available, give 600 mg – 1 g PO/ng loading dose, then 200 mg every 6 hours. If propylthiouracil is not available (you should not wait for 'the pharmacy to get some up to the ward tomorrow') give carbimazole 20 mg, then 20 mg three times daily.

> Lugol's iodine (saturated solution of potassium iodide) – five drops every 6 hours, beginning 4 hours after starting propylthiouracil/carbimazole (not before as thyroid hormone stores may be increased) to inhibit further release of thyroxine.

Supportive measures particular to thyrotoxic crisis

> Hyperpyrexia – peripheral cooling measures and paracetamol. Do not use aspirin as it can displace thyroid hormone from its binding sites.

> Tachycardia – give propranolol 1 mg IV, repeated every 20 minutes as necessary up to total of 5 mg; or give 40–80 mg PO four times daily. Be careful if the patient has cardiac failure. Esmolol, a short acting beta-blocker, can be used as an infusion for immediate management of sympathetic overactivity.

> AF – consider digitalisation, but note that higher doses of digoxin than usual may be needed due to relative resistance to the drug.

> Steroids – eg hydrocortisone 200 mg IV, then 100 mg every 6 hours; or dexamethasone 2 mg PO four times daily.

Treat possible precipitating causes

> Start broad-spectrum antibiotics if there is any suggestion of infection.

1.3.24 Sudden onset of severe headache

Case history

A 34-year-old woman presents to the emergency department with a sudden onset, severe, occipital headache. You are the duty medical doctor on call and are asked to assess her.

Introduction

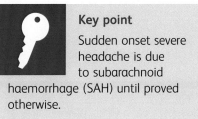

Key point

Sudden onset severe headache is due to subarachnoid haemorrhage (SAH) until proved otherwise.

History of the presenting complaint

Features of the headache to enquire about are:

> Speed of onset – SAHs come on suddenly. Specifically ask how long it took from them first noticing the headache to it being at peak intensity. In SAH this is usually less than 1–2 minutes.

> Severity – patients usually describe the pain of SAH as the worst they have ever had, and often 'like being hit over the head with a baseball bat.'

> Time of onset – headaches that wake from sleep (rather than being noticed on waking) are significant, as are those occurring on exercise – including sexual activity. A sudden severe headache occurring during sexual activity may be a primary headache disorder but a first such presentation should be investigated to exclude SAH.

Have there been any other symptoms such as nausea, vomiting, blurring of vision or any other neurological dysfunction, and did these come on before or after the headache? Did the patient lose consciousness for any period? Migraine is often associated with a visual aura prior to the onset of headache; SAH may give negative symptoms such as loss of consciousness, visual impairment or weakness that follow the headache. Photophobia is a feature of SAH, but also of meningitis and migraine.

Other relevant history

> Does the patient have a history of headaches, and if so, were they similar/different in nature to this? Have a lower threshold for investigating if the patient feels this is not their 'usual' headache or is significantly worse.

> Does the patient smoke or use illicit drugs (amphetamine and cocaine are associated with SAH, as is smoking)?

> Ask about any family history of SAH or related conditions (adult polycystic kidney disease and some connective tissue diseases).

Are there features to support another diagnosis? Have there been any recent problems with the eyes, ears or sinuses that could indicate sinusitis or otitis media? Has the patient travelled abroad recently or had symptoms to suggest infection: could this be meningitis or malaria (see Sections 1.3.25 and 1.3.30)?

Examination

Patients with severe headache range from those who walk into the emergency department to those who are comatose with cardiorespiratory collapse. The general approach to the examination of the patient in coma is discussed in Section 1.3.29, and for the patient with cardiovascular collapse in Section 1.3.2. In dealing with the patient with suspected SAH, aside from assessing and alleviating pain and anxiety, the following are of particular importance:

> Check GCS score (Fig 29) immediately to establish baseline.

> Focal neurological signs – especially pupillary size and reaction. A fixed, dilated pupil is an extremely worrying physical sign in this context, indicating damage to the third cranial nerve either from generalised compression (raised intracranial pressure) or localised compression (aneurysm of the posterior communicating artery).

> Features of SAH – neck stiffness, photophobia, subconjunctival haemorrhages (also a feature of meningococcal disease, but subconjunctival haemorrhages where you cannot see the lateral limits are indicative of SAH) and subhyaloid haemorrhages. Also check for features (much less likely) of connective tissue diseases and for adult polycystic kidney disease which predispose to SAH.

> Features to support another diagnosis – high fever; and infection of ears, nose and throat.

Investigation

The general approach to investigation of the patient in coma is discussed in Section 1.3.29. With regard to general investigations, note that SAH is often associated with cardiac dysfunction:

> The ECG shows ST and T-wave changes in 70–80% of cases, including an infarct pattern in 10–15%.

> The chest radiograph shows either neurogenic or cardiogenic pulmonary oedema developing in 10–15% of patients.

> The serum troponin level is often slightly or moderately elevated.

Computerised tomography brain scan

If SAH is suspected, then unenhanced CT scan is the investigation of choice (Fig 36). The sensitivity for SAH is 98% at 12 hours, falling to 93% at 24 hours. Patients who present some days after onset of symptoms may be difficult to diagnose as the degradation of blood in the subarachnoid space means that it may have the same density as brain tissue.

Lumbar puncture

Patients presenting with a thunderclap headache who have a normal CT scan should undergo lumbar puncture if there are no contraindications (see Section 3.2). This should be performed a minimum of 12 hours after the onset of symptoms: prior to

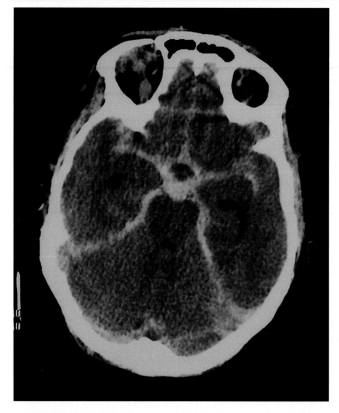

Fig 36 An unenhanced CT scan showing blood outlining the circle of Willis in a patient with a subarachnoid haemorrhage.

this the breakdown products of red cells in the cerebrospinal fluid (CSF) may not be apparent. Opening pressure should be recorded and at least three serial CSF specimens should be examined for xanthochromia and red cell count. CSF should also be sent for spectrophotometry (looking for oxyhaemoglobin or bilirubin).

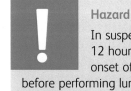

Hazard

In suspected SAH wait 12 hours from the onset of symptoms before performing lumbar puncture to avoid a false-negative result.

Management

All patients with SAH should be discussed with the regional neurosurgical centre unless they are terminally ill from an unrelated cause.

The important features of medical management of aneurysmal SAH are:

> Analgesia – pain will increase the catecholamine response and will potentially increase the risk of rebleeding or cardiac dysfunction.

> Oxygen – all patients should receive high-flow oxygen. There will be a penumbral area around the region of the SAH that is at risk of ischaemic damage.

> Fluid – assuming they have normal renal function and adequate urinary output, patients should receive at least 3 L/day of 0.9% saline. Solutions containing dextrose should be avoided: once the dextrose is consumed the fluid is hypotonic and will preferentially move into cerebral cells, thereby worsening cerebral oedema.

> Nimodipine (a selective calcium channel blocker) reduces the risk of vasospasm and therefore protects against cerebral ischaemia.

Nimodipine 60 mg PO 4-hourly for 3 weeks should be given to all patients with SAH who are not hypotensive (systolic BP <110 mmHg). It can also be given via infusion.

> Bed rest; and stool softeners to avoid excessive straining when opening the bowels.

Further comments

80% of SAHs are due to a ruptured aneurysm while a further 15% are due to arteriovenous malformations.

Major intracerebral complications of subarachnoid haemorrhage

> Rebleeding – the risk of rebleeding from a cerebral aneurysm following acute SAH is about 4% in the first 24 hours and 1%/day thereafter.

> Hydrocephalus – the risk depends on both the volume and site of blood within the subarachnoid space. Large bleeds are more likely to cause hydrocephalus through blockage of the arachnoid granulations responsible for reabsorption of CSF: blood clots situated in narrow areas of the ventricular system, such as the third ventricle or the aqueduct, may cause obstructive hydrocephalus.

> Vasospasm (delayed ischaemic neurological deficit) – generally occurs between 5–12 days after SAH. Breakdown products of blood are thought to trigger vasospasm of nearby arteries, resulting in symptomatic ischaemia that may be irreversible.

Definitive treatments for aneurysmal subarachnoid haemorrhage

CT angiography or catheter angiography is used to identify the site and number of aneurysms. Once identified these can be treated either by endovascular coiling or surgical clipping. If both techniques are available in a given centre, the decision regarding coiling versus clipping depends on the site and nature of the aneurysm, the number of aneurysms present and the comorbidity of the patient.

> Clipping – a surgical clip is placed around the neck of the aneurysm.

> Coiling – a catheter is inserted, usually via a femoral artery, and fed up to site of aneurysm; thrombogenic coils are placed within the aneurysm to secure it.

1.3.25 Severe headache with fever

Case history
A 22-year-old student presents with 24 hours of increasing headache associated with high fever and a rash. Previously he was well. You are the on-call medical doctor and are asked to see him in the emergency department.

Introduction

Key point
This man almost certainly has meningococcal meningitis and septicaemia and must be treated as such immediately.

History of presenting problem

Key point
Before embarking on taking a history the top priority is to determine 'is this patient well, ill, very ill or nearly dead?' If they are the latter, get help from the ICU immediately.

If circumstances permit history taking, then ask about the following:

> Onset of headache – the headache of meningitis is usually a dull, progressively worsening one, in contrast to that of SAH (see Section 1.3.24).

> Systemic features – flu-like symptoms of fever, sweats, muscle aches, joint pains and nausea/vomiting suggest systemic infection and are common in meningitis.

> Photophobia – a common complaint in meningitis but also seen with migraine and SAH. Do not overinterpret this symptom: anyone with a severe headache of any cause will be averse to bright lights.

> Sore throat and earache – these may be the primary cause of the headache or may indicate the source of meningitis.

> Behaviour – recent changes in behaviour might point towards meningoencephalitis.

Other relevant history

Given the immediate working diagnosis of meningococcal meningitis: has the patient been in contact with anyone with meningitis? Are they up to date with their vaccinations? Where do they live, who are their close contacts and have any of these been ill recently? Contacts will need to be traced and appropriate antibiotic prophylaxis given if the case is confirmed as due to meningococcal disease.

It will also be important to ask about whether the patient has received any antibiotics recently, which may prevent successful culture of the organism, and if they have any allergies – especially to penicillin.

Examination

The general approach to the examination of the patient in coma is discussed in Section 1.3.29, and for the patient with cardiovascular collapse in Section 1.3.2. Cases with a high clinical suspicion of meningitis should be in respiratory isolation. In dealing with a case of suspected meningococcal meningitis, note the following.

Skin, mucous membranes and eyes

Any new rash should be treated as highly suspicious: although the rash of meningococcal septicaemia is classically purplish and non-blanching (Fig 37), in its early stages it may be erythematous and macular. Look for infarcts in the nailbeds, resulting from immune complex deposition. Look carefully for subconjunctival and sublingual haemorrhages. Look in the fundi for subhyaloid haemorrhages and papilloedema.

Features of meningeal irritation

Several physical signs are described, the most commonly used being:

> Neck stiffness – there is an involuntary resistance to flexion when the physician attempts to bend the patient's neck such that the chin touches the chest. The best known of several signs attributed to Brudziński is positive when such flexion of the patient's neck causes them to flex both their hips and knees.

> Kernig's sign – the patient lies in bed with their hip and knee flexed; a positive sign is recorded when an attempt by the physician to extend the knee is resisted involuntarily by the patient (and usually causes pain).

Investigation

Hazard
Suspected meningococcal septicaemia – treat first; ask questions afterwards.

The general approaches to investigation of the patient who is very ill or in coma are discussed in Sections 1.3.2 and 1.2.29. In this case the particular emphasis will clearly be on trying to confirm the diagnosis of meningococcal septicaemia/meningitis.

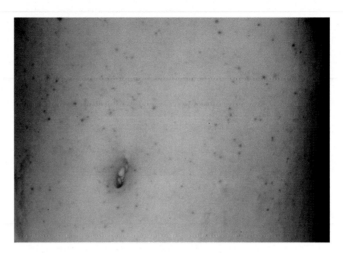

Fig 37 Characteristic petechial rash of meningococcal septicaemia.

Key point
Insert an intravenous cannula, draw blood cultures through it and give intravenous antibiotics.

Neisseria meningitidis can be cultured from blood, scrapings of skin lesions and cerebrospinal fluid (CSF); the diagnosis of meningococcal disease may also be made immunologically. See Section 3.2 for discussion of contraindications, technique and interpretation of the findings of lumbar puncture.

Management

Aside from supportive care, described in Section 1.3.2, the essential requirement is to give an appropriate antibiotic without delay – the choice depends on local sensitivities, but usually high-dose cephalosporin, eg cefotaxime 2 g IV 4-hourly or ceftriaxone 2 g IV 12-hourly. Consideration should be given to adjuvant dexamethasone treatment and where signs of severe sepsis are present the 'Sepsis Six Bundle' should be started.

Further comments

Meningitis is a notifiable disease: refer the case to public health for contact tracing. Household and other intimate contacts are recommended to take prophylactic antibiotics (eg a single dose of ciprofloxacin 750 mg orally) and to be immunised (if meningococcaemia is due to serogroup C or A).

1.3.26 Acute paraparesis

Case history
A 38-year-old woman is referred urgently by her GP. For the last 3 days she has had mild bilateral leg weakness with difficulty climbing stairs. She has not passed urine for 18 hours and is distressed. You are asked to see and assess her.

Introduction

The diagnosis in this case is cord compression until proved otherwise, but consider the possibilities listed in Table 19 as you deal with the case.

History of the presenting problem

Important aspects to explore include:

> Speed of progression – cord compression is usually acute, producing non-progressive and asymmetric weakness. Guillain–Barré syndrome typically presents as a distal weakness – usually with tingling or a tight, 'bound' sensation of the

Table 19	Causes of acute or subacute paraplegia or quadriplegia	
Frequency	**General type of cause**	**Clinical condition**
Common	Cord compression	Primary/secondary tumour
		Herniated disc
	Other	Guillain–Barré syndrome
		Transverse myelitis (idiopathic, MS, SLE, Behçet's and HIV)
Must consider	Vascular causes	Aortic dissection
		Spinal cord SAH
		Thrombosis of anterior spinal artery
	Cord compression	Epidural abscess
		Osteomyelitis (including TB)
	Other	Deficiency diseases (B_{12} deficiency, beriberi and alcoholic neuropathy)
Rare		Toxic polyneuropathies
		Severe hypokalaemia
		Tick paralysis
		Porphyric polyneuropathy

MS, multiple sclerosis; SAH, subarachnoid haemorrhage; SLE, systemic lupus erythematosus; TB, tuberculosis.

distal lower limbs – and progresses steadily over a few days.

> Presence or absence of pain – sudden onset of pain in association with weakness suggests a herniated disc, spinal SAH or aortic dissection with involvement of the spinal arteries.

> Sensory symptoms – these (usually painful) often precede weakness by some days or even weeks in cord compression; in Guillain–Barré syndrome they usually occur simultaneously or slightly later.

> Bladder or bowel involvement – urinary or bowel dysfunction suggests cord compression.

> Associated symptoms – anorexia, malaise and weight loss should raise the possibility of disseminated malignancy. Fever, rigors or sweats suggest osteomyelitis, TB or an epidural abscess.

Hazard

Breathlessness in the patient with paraparesis or quadriparesis is a sinister symptom – respiratory failure can be rapidly progressive in Guillain–Barré syndrome and around a third of patients require ventilatory support.

Other relevant history

A thorough past medical history is crucial: is there any previous history of malignancy, eg breast cancer, or of a multisystem disorder, such as systemic lupus erythematosus (SLE)? Previous neurological symptoms might point to a diagnosis of multiple sclerosis (MS). Intravenous drug usage may lead to osteomyelitis, epidural abscess or (less likely) transverse myelitis in association with HIV infection.

Examination: general features

Poor general health may indicate malignancy, anorexia or nutritional deficiencies. Breast and thyroid examination are important to exclude two malignancies that can metastasise to the spine in this age group.

Cardiovascular abnormalities, eg tachycardia, bradycardia, hypertension or hypotension, may indicate autonomic dysfunction in association with Guillain–Barré syndrome.

Respiratory assessment is especially important in suspected Guillain–Barré syndrome. Can the patient speak in full sentences or only words at a time? A simple method to quantitate respiratory disability is to ask the patient to take a deep breath and then to count out loud as far as they can … 1, 2, 3, 4 etc. This correlates fairly well with forced vital capacity and can be easily reproduced to assess if things are getting better or worse.

Is the patient's bladder palpable? Autonomic involvement may occur in a variety of conditions, including Guillain–Barré syndrome, but the most urgent need is to exclude cord compression. A digital rectal examination to test anal tone is also essential.

Examination: nervous system

Evidence of cord compression

> Motor – below the level of an acute cord compression weakness may be associated with hypotonia, hyporeflexia and unresponsive plantars, but hypertonia, hyperreflexia and upgoing plantars develop rapidly and may be found at presentation in some cases.

> Sensory – examine carefully for a sensory level, possibly suspended, that defines the most caudal location of a spinal lesion that could be responsible for the patient's symptoms and signs. Do not forget to check sensation in the saddle area, impairment suggesting a lesion in the cauda equina.

The finding of neurological signs above the level of a cord lesion clearly indicates that more than one neurological site is affected, eg optic atrophy in a patient with MS, or cerebral and spinal metastases in a patient with disseminated malignancy.

Hazard

Urinary retention is not always due to mechanical outflow obstruction

When performing a rectal examination in a patient with urinary retention, always ask 'can you feel me touching you here?' before you start. Patients with cord compression can present with urinary retention and little in the way of leg weakness.

Key point

Sphincter disturbance, sensory loss in the saddle area, and ankle weakness suggest a cauda equina lesion.

Evidence of Guillain–Barré syndrome

> Motor – lower motor neurone weakness, distal more than proximal, with reduced tone and areflexia. Facial involvement and ophthalmoplegia is found in the Miller Fisher syndrome variant.

> Sensory – glove and stocking sensory loss, which is often mild.

Investigation

Key point

Investigation and treatment of spinal cord compression is an emergency – incomplete lesions with sparing of part of the sensory or motor pathways have a much better prognosis than complete lesions: rarely can function be restored once lost. Discuss cases immediately with radiological colleagues and neurosurgical services.

Imaging of the spine

MRI is the investigation of choice in patients with non-traumatic paraplegia or quadriplegia (Fig 38). Plain radiography of the spine may show an obvious lesion. A CT scan or a myelogram may be indicated in individual patients; but CT scanning may not exclude cord compression and may not show evidence of demyelination, and myelography can cause clinical deterioration in patients with cord compression. Patients with metastatic cord compression need whole spine imaging due to the frequent finding of disease at multiple spinal levels.

Other tests

Routine haematological and biochemical screening tests will be required, with

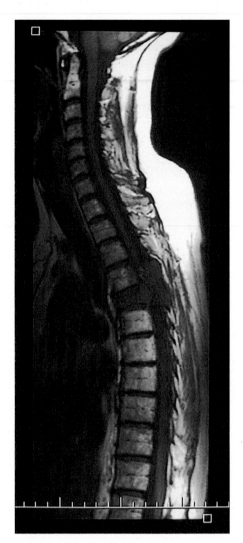

Fig 38 An MRI study (T2-weighted image) showing a spinal secondary deposit causing cord compression.

particular emphasis on looking for evidence of malignancy (anaemia, abnormal liver blood tests, hypercalcaemia, raised inflammatory markers and abnormalities on chest radiography) and – in an older patient – myeloma (serum immunoglobulins, serum protein electrophoresis and urinary Bence Jones proteinuria). Other investigations may be appropriate depending on the clinical context, eg cultures to pursue sepsis/TB and lymph node biopsy.

If Guillain–Barré syndrome is a possibility

This is primarily a clinical diagnosis but can be supported by lumbar puncture (after cord compression excluded by imaging; typically reveals elevated protein with normal cell count), nerve conduction studies (absence or impersistence of F-waves) and anti-GQ1b antibodies (positive in Miller Fisher variant). Check stool culture and serology for *Campylobacter jejuni*, serology for atypical pneumonia and cerebrospinal fluid (CSF) for viral infection.

Because of concern about respiratory or cardiac involvement, check and continue to monitor respiratory function tests (forced expiratory volume at 1 second), arterial blood gas (ABG) and ECG.

Management

Specific treatments will depend on the diagnosis, but the following are important for all patients with acute paraplegia:

> Relieve urinary retention (if present).

> Give adequate analgesia.

> Provide a pressure-relieving mattress and turn the patient over regularly to prevent pressure sores.

> Early institution of bowel care.

Cord compression

Disc protrusion requires surgical decompression. Metastatic disease may be treated with high-dose steroids followed by surgical decompression or radiotherapy, depending on the context. Spinal/epidural abscess requires surgical drainage and appropriate antimicrobials.

Guillain–Barré syndrome

Give intravenous immunoglobulin 0.4 g/kg/day for 5 days. Antiarrhythmic and antihypertensive drugs may be required, but use them with caution and

obtain expert help in dealing with these problems that can arise with autonomic instability. Although these measures are important, supportive care may be required for a protracted period of time in spite of effective treatment.

1.3.27 Status epilepticus

Case history

A man who seems to be about 50 years old has been found collapsed in the street with generalised seizures. He has been fitting continuously for 20 minutes by the time he reaches the emergency department. No past history is available, and no family members or friends are present.

Immediate management

> Assess airway, breathing and circulation, and initiate resuscitation if required (see Sections 1.3.1 and 1.3.2).

> Give high-flow oxygen; apply a pulse oximeter to monitor the oxygen saturation.

> Obtain intravenous access.

> Check finger-prick blood glucose; if <2.5 mmol/L give 50 mL 50% glucose as well as high-potency thiamine (eg Pabrinex or Parentrovite) to patients with poor nutrition.

Hazard

Insertion of an oral airway is almost impossible during a fit and is likely to cause trauma either to the teeth or to the soft tissues if performed – wait until the fit is terminated and then insert an oral or nasal airway as necessary.

Key point

To terminate status epilepticus give:

> lorazepam (4 mg IV at a rate of 2 mg/min): watch for sedation, respiratory depression and hypotension. This terminates fits in 60–90% of patients, *or*

> diazepam (10–20 mg IV at a rate of 5 mg/min): an alternative to lorazepam; can be given rectally at a dose of 10–20 mg (rectal gel) if intravenous access cannot be obtained.

If no response within 10–15 minutes, repeat either of the above medications and if seizures persist then commence:

> phenytoin (15–20 mg/kg IV at a rate of 25–50 mg/min).

> fosphenytoin (15–20 mg phenytoin equivalents/kg IV at a rate of 50–100 phenytoin equivalent/min; fosphenytoin sodium 1.5 mg = phenytoin sodium 1 mg).

For patients already taking phenytoin, the decision on whether to load with phenytoin or call for anaesthetic support will require senior input.

Call for anaesthetic help if there is still no response: the patient may need to be fully anaesthetised using barbiturates or non-barbiturate drugs (eg propofol), intubated and ventilated.

History of the presenting problem

This man is clearly not in a position to give an immediate history, but consider the possibilities shown in Table 20.

Table 20	Causes of status epilepticus	
Common	**Must consider**
Primary epilepsy[1]	Space-occupying lesion
Hypoglycaemia	Anoxia
SAH/CVA	Intracerebral infection and meningitis
Alcohol/drug withdrawal	Other metabolic disturbance, eg hyponatraemia or uraemia
	Pseudoseizures

1 New or established diagnosis, the latter often with non-compliance with medication
CVA, cerebrovascular accident; SAH, subarachnoid haemorrhage.

If the patient remains semi-conscious following termination of his fit then useful information may be obtained from:

> ambulance crew/notes

> medic alert bracelet or necklace – look carefully at any jewellery

> other clues – is he carrying any identification, medication or prescription cards that might suggest he is a known epileptic or diabetic?

> emergency department staff – many patients with epilepsy are regular attenders: does anyone recognise him?

When discussion can take place with the patient or someone who knows them, then for known epileptics it will be important to pursue reasons for the development of their status epilepticus. Have they been taking their medication (some epileptics are reluctant to accept their diagnosis)? Have they had an intercurrent illness that has prevented them from taking their medication or may have altered its absorption (eg gastroenteritis)? Have there been any other changes in their medication that might have altered drug levels? Is there an underlying cause for their epilepsy that is progressing (eg a cerebral space-occupying lesion)? Have they taken large amounts of alcohol or non-prescription drugs that have precipitated the attack?

Examination

The general approach to the examination of the patient in coma is discussed in Section 1.3.29, but particular points to note in this case would be:

> Poor general nutrition or hygiene – may indicate alcohol or drug abuse, or (less likely) disseminated malignancy.

> Signs of chronic liver disease due to alcohol abuse, eg spider naevi, jaundice, Dupuytren's contractures and bruising.

> Signs of drug abuse, eg track marks.

> GCS score and focal neurological signs – pupillary signs and asymmetry of limb movements may be abnormal following a fit, but persistent asymmetry strongly suggests a focal intracranial lesion.

Investigations

The first investigation of the patient presenting with status epilepticus should be measurement of finger-prick blood glucose to exclude hypoglycaemia. The requirement for further investigation will depend on the patient's response to immediate treatment to terminate the fit. The known epileptic who responds rapidly and wakes up to give an account that explains events ('I've stopped taking my tablets') does not require extensive investigation. When this is not the case, consider the following.

Routine tests

Blood tests – laboratory glucose, electrolytes/renal/liver/bone profile (hyponatraemia, hypocalcaemia and hypomagnesaemia can cause fits, as can hepatic encephalopathy or advanced renal failure), FBC, clotting (impairment increases risk of intracerebral haemorrhage) and anticonvulsant levels.

Chest radiograph – may show cause of status, eg malignancy that has metastasised to the brain, or complication, eg aspiration pneumonia.

Urine sample – for drug toxicology testing (may be useful in some cases).

Imaging

CT and/or MRI are warranted in almost all cases of unexplained status epilepticus, but patients should only be moved from the emergency department once they have been stabilised.

Other tests

If there is suspicion of an infective cause then this should be pursued, eg blood cultures, lumbar puncture (if there is no contraindication on CT), thick film for malaria and MRI scanning (Fig 39) as appropriate.

Arterial blood gases (ABGs) can usefully document the adequacy of oxygenation and ventilation, and may also reveal unexpected metabolic acidosis, which gives a clue to poisoning as an explanation for fits, eg ethylene glycol (antifreeze).

Electroencephalography may be required in patients who remain unconscious: fits may become progressively more subtle in prolonged epilepsy (non-convulsive status epilepticus).

Further management

Specific treatment, if possible, will be determined by the cause of the fitting. Patients who are recovering from a seizure should be nursed in the recovery position with appropriate management of their airway (nasopharyngeal or oral airway; suction), continued high-flow oxygen and close monitoring (vital signs, neurological observations, ECG and oxygen saturation) until they

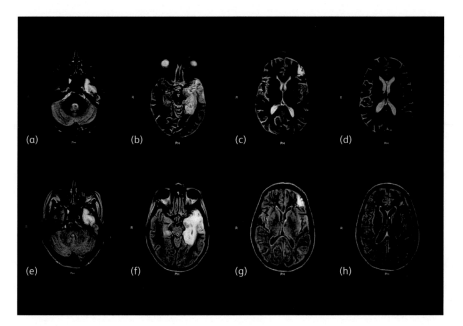

Fig 39 A MRI of herpes simplex encephalitis showing classical cortical distribution mainly in the temporal and parietal lobes: **(a–d)** T2-weighted images; **(e–h)** fluid attenuated inverse response (FLAIR) images.

have recovered fully. A suitable pressure-relieving mattress, intravenous fluids and urinary catheter will be required if they are slow to regain consciousness.

Referral to a neurologist will be required for optimal long-term management of epilepsy in appropriate cases.

1.3.28 Stroke

Case history

A 68-year-old woman is found on the living room floor by her husband. He phones for an ambulance, which brings her to the emergency department where she is immediately observed to have right-sided weakness and slurred speech. She has a long history of poorly controlled hypertension. You are asked to assess her.

Introduction

The working diagnosis must be that this woman has had a stroke, although other conditions must be considered (Table 21).

The most likely diagnosis is an acute stroke. Immediate priorities are:

Resuscitation and immediate assessment

> Airway, breathing and circulation (ABC) – in stroke, aim for an oxygen saturation of 94–98%, or 88–92% if the patient is at risk of hypercapnic respiratory failure.

> Patients with a GCS score <12 may benefit from a nasal or oral airway – those with a GCS score <8 need to be considered for elective intubation.

> Check blood glucose and correct if abnormal.

Diagnosis

Key point

Has the patient had a stroke?

If the Recognition of Stroke in Emergency Room (ROSIER) score (Table 22) suggests that a stroke is likely, then an immediate CT scan should be arranged and the stroke team informed. This is particularly urgent if the patient is within the thrombolysis window and has a significant neurological deficit.

History of the presenting problem

She has some difficulty with speech – described (perhaps loosely) in the scenario as being 'slurred' – and so obtaining a history from her may be difficult. First consider whether or not she has dysphasia.

Key point

Assess whether or not a patient who might have had a stroke is dysphasic before trying to take a history:

> Is their speech fluent?

> Do they have any receptive dysphasia – can they obey a one-, then two-, then three-step command?

> Do they have any expressive dysphasia, eg nominal dysphasia?

If a history can be obtained from the patient or her husband, ask about the following:

> Onset of symptoms – strokes come on suddenly, so a weakness of gradual onset would suggest an alternative diagnosis.

Table 21 Differential diagnosis of stroke

Common	Must consider
Thrombotic stroke	Subdural haematoma
Embolic stroke	Giant cell arteritis
SAH	Hypoglycaemia
	Aortic/carotid dissection
	Encephalitis/meningitis
	Cerebral abscess
	Cerebral tumour
	(primary or secondary)

SAH, subarachnoid haemorrhage.

Table 22 Recognition of Stroke in Emergency Room (ROSIER) assessment tool

Has there been loss of consciousness or syncope?	−1 point
Has there been seizure activity?	−1 point
Is there new acute onset of the following:	
asymmetrical facial weakness	+1 point
asymmetrical arm weakness	+1 point
asymmetrical leg weakness	+1 point
speech disturbance	+1 point
visual field defect / ophthalmoplegia	+1 point

If total score is 1–5 then stroke is likely.
If total score is zero or less then stroke is unlikely.

> Associated symptoms – a sudden severe headache preceding the collapse may suggest a SAH or intracerebral haemorrhage. A history of jaw pain and/or temporal tenderness suggests giant cell arteritis. Has she been pyrexial? If so, consider unusual cerebral pathology such as brain abscess (commonly spread from infection in the sinuses or middle ear) or meningitis.

> Stroke typically results in loss of function, so the presence of positive symptoms (eg tingling/unusual sensations) typically suggests another diagnosis.

Other relevant history

Previous medical history

Have there been any preceding episodes? Ask particularly about amaurosis fugax and transient ischaemic attacks. This woman is hypertensive, but are there any other risk factors for cerebrovascular disease, eg cardiovascular disease, peripheral vascular disease, smoking or diabetes? Is there a history of malignancy that might have led to brain metastasis? You should also ask about bleeding, recent surgery and any contraindications to thrombolysis if this is being considered.

Functional/social history

This woman has only just arrived in the emergency department and a range of outcomes – ranging from rapid resolution of symptoms to permanent disability or death – are possible, but getting a social history is important. What was the patient's previous level of functioning? What is the home like – eg does it have stairs?

Examination

General examination

Examination will focus on the neurological system but there are also important points to note on general examination:

> Temperature – pyrexia could be due to a secondary infection as a result of the stroke (eg pneumonia) or much less likely due to the primary cause of the 'stroke' (eg cerebral abscess).

> Check her pulse: is she in atrial fibrillation (AF)?

> Check her BP – patients are often hypertensive after a stroke, but their cerebral autoregulation is impaired and antihypertensive agents should not be given except in extreme circumstances (see below).

> Cardiovascular – are there any murmurs? Could this be an embolic stroke from endocarditis (look for stigmata)? Are there carotid bruits or other evidence of vascular disease, ie other arterial bruits or absent peripheral pulses? Could there be an aortic dissection (feel both radial pulses and check her BP in both arms if they are not clearly equal)?

> Respiratory – check the adequacy of her ventilation and for evidence of aspiration.

Neurological examination

You should perform a full neurological examination, but it is particularly important to check (and document):

> GCS score – to establish baseline condition.

> Neck stiffness – if present, the diagnosis is likely to be primary SAH.

> Focal signs – to determine the approximate site of the lesion (Table 23).

Investigation

Imaging

Key point

CT scan of the brain (ideally CT perfusion) should be performed as soon as possible (within 12 hours of admission) in all patients with acute stroke, but is particularly urgent (within 1 hour) in patients:

> eligible for thrombolysis

> on anticoagulation or with a known bleeding tendency

> with depressed conscious level

> with severe headache at onset of symptoms

> with papilloedema, neck stiffness or fever on examination

> with unexplained progressive or fluctuating symptoms.

Other routine investigations

Basic investigations should include:

Blood tests – glucose, FBC (note polycythaemia or thrombocytopenia), clotting screen, inflammatory markers (consider giant cell arteritis if these

are grossly elevated without other explanation), electrolytes and liver/bone profiles.

Chest radiograph – looking for aspiration, and occasionally another pathology.

ECG – to look for atrial fibrillation or evidence of recent myocardial infarction (about 5% of myocardial infarctions in older people present with stroke).

Table 23 The Oxfordshire Community stroke subclassification system (also known as the Bamford classification)

Syndrome	Neurological deficit	Cause
TACS	New higher cerebral dysfunction (eg dysphasia, dyscalculia and visuospatial disorder) *and* Homonymous visual field defect *and* Ipsilateral motor and/or sensory deficit involving at least two out of three areas of the face, arm or leg	Large cortical stroke in middle cerebral, or middle and anterior cerebral artery territories
PACS	Two out of the three components of the TACS *or* New higher cerebral dysfunction alone *or* Motor/sensory deficit more restricted than those classified as a LACS (eg isolated hand involvement)	Cortical stroke in middle or anterior cerebral artery territory
LACS	Pure motor stroke *or* Pure sensory stroke *or* Sensorimotor stroke *or* Ataxic hemiparesis *or* Dysarthria and clumsy hand Note that evidence of higher cortical involvement or disturbance of consciousness excludes a lacunar syndrome	Subcortical stroke due to small vessel disease
POCS	Ipsilateral cranial nerve palsy with contralateral motor and/or sensory deficit *or* Bilateral motor and/or sensory deficit *or* Disorder of conjugate eye movement *or* Cerebellar dysfunction without ipsilateral long tract involvement *or* Isolated homonymous visual field defect	Stroke in posterior circulation, brainstem or cortex

LACS, lacunar syndrome; PACS, partial anterior circulation syndrome; POCS, posterior circulation syndrome; TACS, total anterior circulation syndrome.

Management

Key point

The priorities in management of all patients with acute brain injury are to minimise secondary brain damage and maximise potential recovery.

Immediate management

> Airway, breathing and circulation (ABC) – supplemental oxygen should be given if saturations are <95% on air. Patients with a GCS score <12 may benefit from a nasal or oral airway; those with a GCS score <8 need to be considered for elective intubation.

> Obtain intravenous access and give intravenous fluids until the patient's swallow has been assessed as safe; treat hypoglycaemia promptly.

> Swallowing should be assessed using a swallow screening test. If there are any concerns about safety of swallowing then they should be kept nil by mouth and referred for formal assessment.

> Consider thrombolysis (only if there is an agreed hospital protocol and staff experienced in its use).

> Aspirin 300 mg once daily (by nasogastric (NG) tube or rectally if swallowing concerns) should be started 24 hours after thrombolysis or as soon as possible after exclusion of intracerebral haemorrhage in patients not receiving thrombolysis.

> BP control in patients with severe hypertension who are candidates for thrombolysis. This is normally using intravenous labetalol. If BP remains over 185/110 mmHg after two doses of labetalol then thrombolysis is contraindicated.

Key point

Can the patient with a stroke eat and drink?

The presence of a gag reflex is a poor guide to safe swallowing and hence a formal swallow assessment by trained staff is essential. Fluids are more difficult to swallow than semisolids.

Thrombolysis in acute stroke

Key point

Patients with acute ischaemic stroke should be considered for thrombolysis if they have a significant neurological deficit and fulfil the following criteria:

> intracranial haemorrhage excluded on imaging

> definite time of onset within last 3–4.5 hours (thrombolysis must be administered as soon as possible within 4.5 hours from symptom onset).

The severity of symptoms should also be considered. This can be assessed objectively using the National Institutes of Health Stroke Scale (NIHSS). Patients with mild symptoms, or those whose symptoms are rapidly improving, are unlikely to benefit from thrombolysis.

Hazard

Contraindications to thrombolysis in acute stroke:

> rapidly improving neurological condition

> time of onset unknown

> seizure at onset

> arterial puncture at a non-compressible site or lumbar puncture within last 7 days

> major surgery within last 14 days

> gastrointestinal or urinary tract haemorrhage within 21 days

> head injury, intracranial surgery or stroke within last 3 months

> any history of intracranial haemorrhage, brain tumour, intracranial arteriovenous malformation or aneurysm

> BP >185/110 mmHg after treatment

> warfarin with international normalised ratio (INR) >1.7, other anticoagulation (full-dose low-molecular-weight heparin, rivaroxaban, dabigatran)

> platelets <100 × 10^9/L

> hypoglycaemia or hyperglycaemia.

Patients who have received thrombolysis should be admitted to an acute stroke unit and monitored closely for possible complications. In the event of neurological deterioration consider urgent CT scan to exclude intracranial haemorrhage.

Continuing management
All patients with an acute stroke should ideally be admitted to a specialist acute stroke unit for initial management and rehabilitation.

> General care – nurse on a pressure-relieving mattress; a urinary Conveen or catheter may be required; full-length thromboembolic disease stockings should be applied to prevent DVT, along with early mobilisation if possible.

> All patients should have their swallowing function screened and be referred for formal assessment of swallowing if there are concerns. Patients who are unable to swallow should be fed through a nasogastric tube until it is safe to resume oral food and fluids.

> Glycaemic control – good glycaemic control improves the outcome from acute stroke; aim to maintain blood glucose between 4 and 11 mmol/L, if necessary using a variable rate intravenous insulin infusion.

> Continue aspirin 300 mg daily for 2 weeks. If patients have a history of dyspepsia then give aspirin with a proton pump inhibitor. Patients who are allergic to aspirin should be given an alternative antiplatelet agent.

> Early referral to speech therapy, physiotherapy and occupational therapy.

Blood pressure control in acute stroke

Hazard

Immediate attempts to lower the pressure are much more likely to do harm than good: cerebral autoregulation is disturbed and rapid reduction of BP may reduce cerebral perfusion below a critical threshold.

BP commonly increases following acute stroke and settles over the next 24–48 hours. Only start antihypertensive treatment in patients with acute stroke if BP is consistently above 220/120 mmHg or there is a hypertensive emergency (hypertensive encephalopathy, hypertensive nephropathy, hypertensive cardiac failure or MI, aortic dissection, pre-eclampsia or intracerebral haemorrhage). In this circumstance labetalol is a reasonable first choice, aiming to reduce the BP by 10–15% in the first 24 hours.

Secondary prevention
Patients who have had a stroke are at high risk of further events. The following points should be considered during their admission:

> BP control – aiming for BP <140/90 mmHg in the long term (after the acute phase).

> Lipid-lowering therapy with a statin (eg simvastatin 40 mg daily).

> Antiplatelets – first-line treatment is clopidogrel 75 mg monotherapy. If this is not tolerated, then aspirin 75 mg daily and dipyridamole 200 mg twice daily can be used in combination.

> Anticoagulation – patients in AF should be treated with aspirin 300 mg for 2 weeks, with anticoagulation commenced after this period.

> Carotid artery imaging and carotid endarterectomy if indicated.

> Lifestyle modification – advice on smoking cessation, diet, exercise and alcohol consumption.

Further comments
Depending on the outcome from the stroke, further investigation may be appropriate for selected cases. In young stroke patients make sure that you obtain an accurate drug/social history

(amphetamine and cocaine), consider detailed thrombophilia testing (eg lupus anticoagulant) and pursue possible cardiac sources of emboli (transthoracic and transoesophageal echocardiography).

Haemorrhagic stroke
Patients with haemorrhagic stroke who are on anticoagulation prior to their stroke should have the anticoagulant effect reversed. Monitor for any signs of neurological deterioration and consider neurosurgical referral.

1.3.29 Coma

Case history

A man of about 40 years who lives alone has not been seen for 2 days. His neighbours go to his house to investigate, find him collapsed and call an emergency ambulance. The paramedics give oxygen, obtain venous access and bring him to the emergency department where you are asked to assess him. He is unconscious. The neighbours have not accompanied him to hospital.

Immediate management
In the first 5 minutes of dealing with an unconscious patient the priorities are:

> Assess and manage airway, breathing, circulation (ABC) – if the main problem is with A, B or C, then proceed as described in Sections 1.3.1 and 1.3.2.

> Give high-flow oxygen; apply pulse oximeter to monitor oxygen saturation.

> Obtain intravenous access (if not already established).

> Consider hypoglycaemia – check finger-prick blood glucose and if <2.5 mmol/L give 10% or 20% dextrose IV (see Section 1.3.19).

> Consider opioid toxicity – check pupils and respiratory rate: if the pupils are small and the respiratory rate is low then give 400 µg naloxone IV stat, repeated up to a total of 1.2 mg if there is a response.

> Check temperature – is the patient hypothermic? Always use a low-reading thermometer and measure the rectal temperature (axillary, skin, tympanic and oral temperatures are often inaccurate in this setting). If the patient is hypothermic, start rewarming.

> Check GCS score (Fig 29) and look for localising neurological signs: facial asymmetry; movement of right arm and leg compared to left arm and leg; size and reaction of pupils; and abnormal eye position, gaze or eye movements.

> Consider Wernicke's encephalopathy, especially if there are signs of alcohol abuse, and if this is a possibility give thiamine intravenously (see Section 1.3.16).

Key point

Check finger-prick blood glucose immediately in any patient in coma.

Hazard

The half-lives of most opioids are longer than that of naloxone – patients in coma from opioid overdose often require repeated doses of naloxone or an infusion.

History of the presenting problem

The unconscious patient will clearly not be able to give a history, but consider the diagnoses listed in Table 24 as you gather information from any source that you can.

Table 24 Differential diagnosis of coma

Frequency	Condition
Common	Hypoglycaemia Opioid toxicity Head injury Postictal SAH Stroke Alcohol
Less common/rare	Other poisoning – benzodiazepine, tricyclic antidepressant or carbon monoxide Other intracranial haemorrhage – extradural or subdural Hypothermia Metabolic – hyponatraemia, hepatic encephalopathy or advanced renal failure Infective – encephalitis, meningitis or malaria Non-convulsive status

Frequency is as in UK practice; head injury is usually obvious, but not always.
SAH, subarachnoid haemorrhage.

Details of the precise circumstances at the scene where the patient was found are required, either from the ambulance crew (or their written notes) or from the neighbours if they subsequently come to the hospital; also, any information about the patient's general health / past medical history is very important. Are they known to have diabetes or epilepsy, or any other major medical problem? Are they known to take any regular medications? Where were they found? If at the foot of the stairs, it would suggest a fall. Were there any drug bottles or syringes nearby? What was the state of the surroundings? Was the house well kept? Was there any suggestion of carbon monoxide poisoning? Had a suicide note been left?

Examination

Look for the following in particular after initiating the immediate management described above.

Head-to-toe screen

> General condition – poor nutrition or hygiene may indicate alcohol or drug abuse in this context.

> Signs of chronic liver disease – likely to be due to alcohol abuse.

> Signs of drug abuse, eg track marks.

> Signs of trauma – either as a primary cause of the collapse (feel the back of the head and neck for bruising/ induration) or as a consequence of it (check for features of pressure necrosis and compartment syndromes).

> Respiratory pattern – Cheyne–Stokes respiration is associated with bilateral cortical damage; hyperventilation may occur secondary to metabolic acidosis, pulmonary pathology or – rarely – with brain stem pathology; bizarre respiratory patterns may be associated with brain stem pathology.

Neurological

> Pupillary size and reaction – bilateral fixed and dilated pupils suggest severe damage and are a very poor prognostic sign (but ensure the patient is not wearing cosmetic contact lenses). A unilateral, fixed and dilated pupil

indicates a third nerve lesion, commonly due to uncal herniation from a supratentorial mass lesion or a posterior communicating artery aneurysm. A unilateral Horner's syndrome suggests damage to the hypothalamus or a lateral medullary syndrome. Bilateral, small pupils suggest opioid overdose or more rarely pontine damage.

> Eye movements – abnormal conjugate deviation suggests intracerebral damage. Disconjugate deviation implies damage to cranial nerves III, IV or VI.

> Asymmetry of spontaneous movement of arms/legs or of peripheral tone or reflexes suggests focal neurological damage.

Investigations

Glucose and imaging

The first investigation in the unconscious patient should always be a finger-prick blood glucose. If the patient's GCS score is falling – indicating that they are deteriorating – or there are focal neurological signs, then the next priority is to organise an urgent CT scan of the brain, which may reveal something that requires immediate neurosurgical attention.

Hazard

Do not send a patient in coma for a CT scan without ensuring that their ABC are secure and that they have a suitably experienced member of staff to accompany them.

Other routine tests

FBC, clotting, electrolytes, laboratory glucose and a renal/liver/bone profile may give indication of some of the conditions listed in Table 24. Perform a chest radiograph to rule out aspiration. ECG – about 80% of patients who have had a SAH have ECG changes, which in around 10% suggest an acute MI (AMI).

Other tests in selected cases

Blood cultures will be appropriate if there is clinical suspicion of sepsis, and thick films for malaria are necessary in cases with the possibility of exposure. Lumbar puncture may be required, after CT, in selected patients. Aside from confirming oxygenation and ventilation, ABGs may show metabolic acidosis – a critical clue to the fact that a patient's coma is due to poisoning (see Section 1.3.33).

Management

Specific management will clearly depend on the cause of coma, and you should have a low threshold for treating unlikely but plausible treatable causes, eg giving aciclovir if herpes simplex encephalitis is possible.

Patients who remain in coma after initial resuscitation measures have been undertaken will require transfer to an ICU. Those who recover to a GCS score of ≥8 may be managed in a suitable high-dependency area; there they should be nursed in the recovery position with appropriate management of their airway (nasopharyngeal or oral airway, suction) and continued high-flow oxygen until they have recovered fully, along with ECG and oxygen saturation monitoring and regular neurological and systemic observations. A suitable pressure-relieving mattress, intravenous fluids and a urinary Conveen/catheter will be required.

1.3.30 Fever in a returning traveller

Case history

A 25-year-old man is brought to the emergency department by his friends. He has recently returned from a backpacking trip around Thailand and has not been well since his return. He is drowsy and has a temperature of 39°C. You are asked to review him immediately on his arrival.

Introduction

Malaria

Key point

> Consider malaria in *any* patient presenting to hospital with coma and/or fever and a relevant travel history.

> There are no diagnostic findings on examination.

> Missing the diagnosis can be fatal.

Malaria must be the working diagnosis in this man. Falciparum malaria is usually the cause of severe, complicated malaria. Cerebral malaria, a complication of *Plasmodium falciparum* infection, may present with coma. There will probably be an antecedent history of a short, febrile illness with rigors and headache. Patients infected with *Plasmodium vivax*, *Plasmodium ovale* or *Plasmodium malariae* tend to have milder symptoms. The incubation period is at least 7 days, but remember that vivax and ovale malaria can cause symptoms for the first time more than 12 months after infection.

Other diagnoses

The diagnosis is malaria! However, be wary – Gram-negative sepsis commonly coexists with malaria and typhoid in particular must be considered. Meningitis may be the only manifestation of typhoid, when it may resemble any other pyogenic meningitis. Consider a broad differential including fungal, viral and other protozoal infections. Also consider encephalitis and cerebral abscess, and drug ingestion may be complicating the picture.

History of the presenting problem

This man may be too unwell to give a lucid account, but if he is able to then – aside from routine enquiry about how the illness began, how it progressed, localising symptoms and past medical history – the most important issues in this case are clearly to get a full travel and social history to establish which pathogens the patient may have been exposed to, and whether precautions to prevent infection have been taken. Ask about:

> countries visited, and when

> areas visited – were they rural or urban, rainforest or savannah?

> accommodation used – a useful guide is to ask about the 'star' rating of this

> activities while there, eg freshwater exposure, trekking or healthcare charity work

> dietary exposures – tap water, shell fish etc

> exposure to animals

> sexual history

> vaccinations received prior to travel

> antimalarial chemoprophylaxis and compliance.

Hazard

Malaria can cause misleading localising features such as abdominal pain, diarrhoea, breathlessness or jaundice.

Hazard

The fact that a patient has taken malaria prophylaxis does not rule out malaria – it is 70–90% effective (if taken).

Examination

The general approaches to investigation of the patient who is very ill or in coma are discussed in Sections 1.3.2 and 1.3.29. Malaria produces no diagnostic physical signs. Anaemia and slight jaundice are common, with moderate tender hepatosplenomegaly. There is no rash or lymphadenopathy.

Investigations

An immediate thick and thin malaria film is required (Fig 40). Remember that a single negative film does not rule out malaria: it is very unlikely if three films are negative, although cannot be completely excluded until another diagnosis is made or the illness resolves. Rapid diagnostic tests, which work by detecting malarial antigens in the blood, are increasingly in use as a first-line test. Although even if the rapid diagnostic tests are positive a formal thick and thin film is still required to provide parasite count.

The approach to investigation of the patient who is very ill and/or has suspected sepsis are described in Sections 1.3.2 and 1.3.25. Note that anaemia, leukopenia, thrombocytopenia, abnormal clotting, renal failure and deranged liver function may all be seen with malaria.

Management

Key point

Seek expert advice sooner rather than later.

The general approaches to management of the patient who is very ill or in coma are discussed in

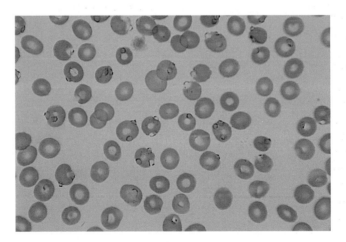

Fig 40 Malaria film showing falciparum malaria.

Sections 1.3.2 and 1.3.29. With regard to the patient with malaria note the following:

> Hypoglycaemia is common in severe malaria – monitor blood glucose hourly and give intravenous dextrose if necessary.

> Remember that there is a clear association between bacterial infection and malaria – in addition to treatment for malaria, treat the patient empirically with broad-spectrum antibiotics after taking blood cultures if they are seriously ill.

Drug treatment of malaria
Falciparum malaria

If the patient can swallow, has no complications, and a parasite count of less than 2%, first-line treatment is now Riamet (each tablet contains artemether 20 mg with lumefantrine 120 mg), four tablets twice daily for 3 days. The 'standard' alternative, which remains the treatment of choice in many countries, is quinine 600 mg (of salt) three times daily for 7 days, followed by a single dose of three tablets of Fansidar (sulfadoxine/pyrimethamine) or doxycycline 100 mg daily for 7 days.

If the patient cannot swallow, has complications, or a parasite count of greater than 2%, then new guidelines are to give intravenous artesunate, which is unlicensed in UK but available in many centres. If there is a delay in obtaining artesunate then start alternative therapy immediately using intravenous quinine sulphate (loading dose 20 mg/kg of dihydrochloride salt, max 1,400 mg, over 4 hours; then 10 mg/kg over 4 hours twice daily). Omit the loading dose of quinine if the patient has received mefloquine within

the last week or quinine has been given in the last 24 hours.

While the quinine is being administered make sure that the patient is on a cardiac monitor and the finger-prick blood glucose is measured hourly.

Vivax, ovale and malariae malaria
Give oral chloroquine 600 mg immediately, followed after 6 hours by 300 mg and then two further doses of 300 mg at 24 and 48 hours intervals. In vivax and ovale infections, chloroquine should then be followed by a 2-week course of primaquine, 15 mg daily, to eliminate parasites from the liver.

Hazard
Remember to screen patients for glucose-6-phosphate dehydrogenase deficiency before giving primaquine or chloroquine otherwise severe haemolysis may ensue.

1.3.31 Anaphylaxis

Case history
A 40-year-old woman has been admitted to the ward for treatment of a community-acquired pneumonia. Shortly after taking the first dose of amoxicillin she complains of difficulty breathing and of swollen lips and tongue. The nurses have put out a 'cardiac arrest' call. You are the leader of the cardiac arrest team and are expected to manage the patient.

Introduction

Key point
Anaphylaxis is a severe allergic reaction to an allergen that the patient has previously been exposed to. It is mediated by antigen-specific cross-linking of immunoglobulin (Ig) E molecules on the surface of tissue mast cells and peripheral blood basophils.

Anaphylactoid reactions are an immediate systemic reaction that mimic anaphylaxis but are not mediated by IgE and may occur on first exposure to the allergen.

Immediate management
This woman is clearly having an anaphylactic reaction:

> Remove or stop possible trigger.

> Assess ABC – airway, breathing and circulation.

> Give high-flow oxygen via a reservoir bag and apply a pulse oximeter to monitor oxygen saturation.

> Give epinephrine (adrenaline) if there is stridor, wheeze, respiratory distress or clinical signs of shock: the initial dose is 0.5 mL 1/1000 solution IM (ie 500 µg), repeated every 5 minutes if there is no sign of improvement.

> Obtain intravenous access.

> Give chlorpheniramine 10 mg IM or IV.

> Give hydrocortisone 200 mg IV.

> Give salbutamol 5–10 mg by nebuliser if bronchospasm is present.

> Give 1 L 0.9% saline stat if the patient is hypotensive.

> Consider nebulised adrenaline 5 mg in 5 mL (5 ampoules of 1:1000) for persistent stridor/bronchospasm.

History of the presenting problem

In this case the history of exposure to a precipitant is clear cut and it is extremely unlikely that the diagnosis is anything other than an anaphylactic reaction to amoxicillin, although the patient may also have received other drugs during their admission. However, in many instances of anaphylaxis it is not clear what the precipitant is, in which case the following issues are important to discuss:

> Is there a previous history of allergy or anaphylaxis?

> Exactly what allergen has precipitated the attack? Many different substances can precipitate anaphylaxis so it is necessary to talk through events in the hour or so preceding the attack in minute detail. Ask 'what have you eaten and drunk? ... anything new? ... any nuts/shellfish (a common precipitant)?; have you been bitten or stung by anything?; have you been exposed to rubber (latex)?; what medications are you taking (salicylates and ACE inhibitors being the most likely culprits)? ... and have there been any recent changes to these? ... and have you taken any non-prescription drugs from any source?'

> Is there a family history of allergy/anaphylaxis (consider C1-inhibitor deficiency)?

Examination, investigation and further management

The approach to the examination, investigation and management of the patient who is extremely ill is discussed in Sections 1.3.1 and 1.3.2, but note the following with regard to the patient with anaphylaxis:

> Serum mast-cell tryptase – elevated following anaphylaxis and useful to confirm the diagnosis when there is clinical doubt. Take three samples at 1) time of event, 2) 1–2 hours after the event, and 3) 24 hours after the event or in the follow-up clinic.

Patients should always be admitted for observation, even if they show an initial good response to treatment. Problems can recur several hours later, especially following ingestion of an allergen or an insect bite.

Further comments

Note that exercise (exercise-induced anaphylaxis) or hot or cold weather can also trigger anaphylaxis in certain patients.

Patients with anaphylaxis should be referred to an allergy clinic for further tests. This may help to identify the allergen, and they may need instruction on the use of self-administered epinephrine (adrenaline – EpiPen).

1.3.32 Back pain

Case history

A 35-year-old man presents with acute low back pain. This came on while lifting up his 3-year-old son and has now been present for 2 days. On getting dressed today he experienced a sudden onset of severe pain and has since been unable to move. He called an ambulance and has been brought to the medical admissions unit where you have been asked to assess him.

Introduction

Back pain is very common and not usually caused by sinister disease, but you must be aware of 'red flags' and pursue appropriate investigation if these are present. If they are not, then you should not investigate unnecessarily but reassure the patient and provide effective analgesia.

History of the presenting problem

Simple mechanical back pain
This typically affects the lower back and can be referred to the buttocks and thighs; it varies with posture or activity and alters over time in response to altered activities or treatment. The referred pain is usually dull and poorly localised; it can affect both legs.

Nerve root or radicular pain
This is usually the patient's main complaint when present. It is sharp and well localised, following a dermatome quite closely; and it is often associated

with sensations of numbness or tingling. Nerve root pain at the common L5 and S1 levels usually extends to the foot or toes.

'Sciatica' is a lay term for pain and sensations of tingling that travel into the buttocks, back of the thigh and into the calf and heel. These symptoms are caused by irritation of the sciatic nerve. Non-specific pain from the lumbar area can also be referred in the distribution of the sciatic nerve.

Red flags

It is essential to check for 'red flags', which increase the chance of the diagnosis being something other than simple mechanical low back pain.

> **Hazard**
> 'Red flags' in the patient with back pain:

> age under 20 or over 55 years

> history of malignancy, steroids, intravenous drug use, HIV or other significant past history

> systemic symptoms such as fever or weight loss

> progressive neurological deficit, eg saddle anaesthesia, sphincteric disturbance, other motor or sensory deficits

> structural deformity

> persistent night pain

> thoracic pain.

Examination

A screening general examination will be required, but attention will properly focus on examination of the back and for neurological signs in the legs. But beware of the patient with back pain who looks ill with evidence of circulatory compromise – they may have a leaking abdominal aortic aneurysm.

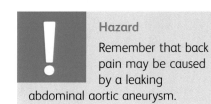

> **Hazard**
> Remember that back pain may be caused by a leaking abdominal aortic aneurysm.

The back

Look for deformity or local tenderness of the back, and perform the passive straight leg raise test (PSLT) for diagnosing nerve root pain due to herniated discs (for which it has high sensitivity (about 90%) but low specificity (about 20%)). With the person lying flat on their back with both legs straight, raise one leg until limited by pain and/or tight hamstrings. Slightly lower the leg to provide relief. In this position, increase tension on the sciatic nerve by dorsiflexion of the foot (or flexion of the neck/compression of the nerve in the popliteal fossa). This will aggravate or elicit pain radiating down the raised leg if there is nerve root irritation. The pain should be relieved by flexion of the knee. The PSLT can also be performed in the sitting position. A discrepancy with the supine PSLT suggests that the symptoms could be factitious.

Neurological examination

Look for focal signs as shown in Table 25.

> **Key point**
> Cauda equina syndrome is due to compression of the cauda equina below the level of L2. This is characterised by urinary and faecal incontinence, urinary retention, sexual dysfunction, saddle anaesthesia and bilateral numbness or weakness in lower limbs (lower motor neuron (LMN) weakness but the precise pattern will vary depending on the level of compression).

Investigation

Imaging

Plain radiological films are unhelpful in the acute setting in the absence of red flags or significant fracture risk; MRI is the best test for diagnosing nerve root compression, discitis and neoplasms (Fig 41).

Other investigations

Patients with simple mechanical back pain should not be investigated. If red flags are present, then investigation should be determined based on clinical suspicion:

> Infection – blood cultures, FBC and inflammatory markers; also diagnostic biopsy.

Table 25	Sensory and motor deficits of root lesions in the leg		
Lesion	Sensory deficit	Motor deficit	Tendon jerks
L2	Often none (across upper thigh)	Hip flexion	No defect
L3	Often none (across lower thigh)	Knee extension	Knee jerk reduced/absent
L4	Medial leg	Foot inversion	Knee jerk reduced/absent
L5	Dorsum of foot	Toe dorsiflexion	No defect
S1	Behind lateral malleolus	Foot plantarflexion and eversion	Ankle jerk reduced/absent

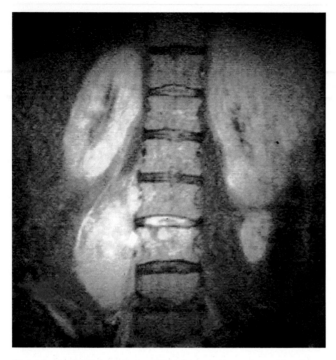

Fig 41 An MRI from a patient presenting with a short history of back pain and perianal anaesthesia. The body of L3 and the right psoas muscle are infiltrated. Biopsy revealed high-grade non-Hodgkin's lymphoma.

> Malignancy – FBC, inflammatory markers, liver/bone profile, prostate-specific antigen and serum immunoglobulins/serum protein electrophoresis/urinary Bence Jones proteins; chest radiograph and bone scan; and diagnostic biopsy.

> Inflammatory – FBC, inflammatory markers, autoimmune rheumatic serology and human leukocyte antigen-B27

Key point

Only consider diagnostic imaging and other investigations if red flags are present or there is significant fracture risk (owing to trauma, steroids or osteoporosis).

Management

Simple mechanical back pain:

> Pharmacological therapy: regular paracetamol should be the initial treatment with addition of an NSAID (with proton pump inhibitor (PPI) protection if over 45) or a weak opioid (eg codeine) if required. Strong opioids can be considered for short-term use if the pain is not controlled and muscle relaxants (eg diazepam 2 mg three times daily) can also be used in the early stages. Consider adding a tricyclic antidepressant (eg amitriptyline), which should be started at a low dose and gradually up titrated.

> Advise patients that it is best to stay physically active

> The prognosis for simple mechanical back pain is good: 90% recover at 6 weeks, although recurrence is common. The prognosis for those with nerve root pain ('sciatica') is less good, with only 50% recovering at 6 weeks.

For those who do not have simple mechanical back pain, specific management will depend on the cause.

Key point

Anyone with symptoms suggestive of cauda equina syndrome needs immediate referral for imaging and (if confirmed) for surgical decompression – this is a surgical emergency.

1.3.33 Self-harm

Case history

A 25-year-old woman is brought to the emergency department following an overdose of 30 x 500 mg paracetamol tablets 9 hours prior to her arrival in hospital. She refuses to say anything other than that she wants to be left alone to die. She has refused all medical intervention. You are asked to see her.

Introduction

Can you treat the patient?

It is common for patients who have intentionally harmed themselves to refuse to stay in hospital or accept treatment. The capacity to consent to medical treatment or make a valid refusal is a legal concept, not a medical one; and therefore it is independent of the diagnosis. If this woman is assumed to have full capacity to refuse medical treatment she may well develop liver failure and possibly die. If a patient has such a capacity, it is of no consequence whether or not you agree with their decision, and whatever their reasons you must respect their decision unless they are detained under the Mental Health Act.

It is reasonable to call on psychiatric services to make an assessment of a patient's capacity, but there is often insufficient time to do this and you therefore must be able to make this assessment as well. Case law has widely recognised that factors such as drugs, fatigue, panic, pain, shock and confusion will erode a patient's capacity, in which case you will be able to proceed with urgent treatment in good faith – provided you are acting in the patient's best interests and in line with the view of a responsible body of medical opinion. Also see Section 1.3.34.

Key point

Treating a patient who does not want to be treated

If you believe that a patient who has taken an overdose has a mental illness and assess that their capacity is in doubt, your duty of care to them allows you to treat them against their will and potentially save their life.

History of the presenting problem

Getting a reliable history from a patient who has taken an overdose can be difficult if not impossible, but to be able to judge the likely medical consequences of an overdose it is clearly necessary to try to establish what has been taken and when. Always presume that other tablets or alcohol have been taken.

Other relevant history

Details of previous medical, psychiatric and social history are required, the main aim of psychiatric assessment being to establish the risk of suicide.

Psychiatric and social background

Is there a past history of deliberate self-harm? Is the patient known to suffer from affective disorder, schizophrenia, alcoholism or drug dependence? Is she socially isolated or recently separated? Have there been any other recent adverse life events? Is there a history of aggressive or impulsive behaviour?

Assessing the risk of suicide

Did she take the overdose on impulse, or had she planned it for some time?

Features that would suggest planning and a high suicide risk include hoarding of pills, taking precautions to make sure that she was alone and undisturbed when she took the pills, leaving a suicide note, giving away treasured possessions before the event; arranging for children to be sent away and the use of more than one means to try and kill herself.

Key point

High risk clinical factors for suicide:

> severe insomnia
> self-neglect
> memory impairment
> agitation
> panic attacks
> pessimism, anhedonia, despair and morbid guilt.

! **Hazard**

> Patients are not experts in pharmacology – do not assume that a small overdose of a relatively safe drug implies lack of lethal intent.

> The degree of suicidal intent can fluctuate.

> Gravely suicidal patients can deliberately conceal their intentions – the patient may appear misleadingly calm after they have made a firm but undisclosed plan to kill themselves.

Examination

The immediate priority in any patient presenting with deliberate self-harm is physical examination, beginning with airway, breathing and circulation (ABC) and the Glasgow Coma Score (GCS). The approach to the patient who is in

circulatory collapse or unconscious is described in Sections 1.3.2 and 1.3.29.

When it is possible to examine the mental state the most important aspects are:

> Does she exhibit self-neglect, anhedonia, pessimism, guilt, remorse and self-recrimination?

> Does she convey a feeling of helplessness and despair?

> Are there depressive or nihilistic delusions?

> Has she experienced command hallucinations?

> Does she wish that she had not survived the overdose?

Investigation

Check levels of paracetamol and salicylate in addition to a routine screen of FBC, clotting, electrolytes and renal/liver/bone profile, with other tests if clinically indicated. Urine and serum samples may need to be saved for later toxicological analysis. Check arterial blood gases (ABGs) if the patient is very unwell, has a GCS score <10 or if ventilation is clinically inadequate.

Management

If the patient is in circulatory shock then resuscitate as described in Section 1.3.2, and if they have impairment of consciousness then as described in Section 1.3.29. For details of specific management of paracetamol toxicity see Section 2.1.2.

Further comments

Risk of suicide

Patients who present with self-harm are 100 times more at risk of suicide compared to the general population. The medical seriousness of an episode is not necessarily indicative of the suicide risk (although violent methods such as attempted shooting are obviously high risk). Self-harm is the most powerful single predictor for completed suicide.

1.3.34 Violence and aggression

Case history

Police have brought a 32-year-old man to the emergency department because they think him disturbed and a risk to others. He is now aggressive and threatening violence towards hospital staff. You are called to assess him.

Introduction

Common law

Key point

Any patient lacking the capacity to consent can be treated under common law.

Nothing can be done for a patient without their consent unless you, as a registered medical practitioner, have assessed and documented them as not having the capacity to consent to treatment. The capacity to consent to or refuse medical treatment requires the patient to understand what is happening, why it is happening and what may happen if they refuse treatment, and that they can retain this information and can make a free decision. Any patient thought to be lacking the capacity to consent can be treated under the common law.

Common law imposes a duty of care on all professional staff to all persons within the hospital. An individual undertakes to provide proper care to those needing it when taking up a professional appointment in a hospital; hence you as a doctor must act in the best interests of the patient.

The Mental Health Act 1983

Key point

The Mental Health Act does not apply to the treatment of physical illness.

The Mental Health Act allows for the legal detention and treatment of adults with mental illness, mental impairment and psychopathic disorder where their admission and/or treatment are considered necessary in the interests of health and safety, for the protection of others and where they are unable to consent to admission and/or treatment.

The Mental Health Act does not apply to the treatment of physical illness, which requires either informed consent from the individual or treatment under common law. The issues can become difficult when physical illness may have led to a disability of the mind through disordered brain function (for example, delirium): this area is not always clear cut. The senior doctor in the department must be involved and a referral made to the psychiatric team as urgently as possible whenever there is consideration of the Mental Health Act being used. Any use of the Mental Health Act will inevitably take time – for arrival of the appropriate personnel and for their subsequent assessment – so usually the detention of the patient will be under common law.

Section 136

Section 136 of the Mental Health Act empowers a police officer to detain and take to a place of safety an individual who may require assessment and/or treatment. In many areas the designated place of safety is a police cell, but some hospital emergency departments may be so designated –

although most are ill-equipped to deal with disturbed individuals (and should resist taking on this role if they do not have adequate facilities). However, the police will bring any person to the emergency department if they consider that the individual might be medically unfit.

Key point

Medical/psychiatric causes of violence and aggression:

> Acute confusional state – an acute, transient, fluctuating, potentially reversible, organic brain disorder characterised by globally impaired consciousness and inattention.

> Psychiatric conditions – most commonly personality disorder and substance abuse.

> Other organic brain pathologies.

History of the presenting problem

Hazard

Dealing with a patient who could be dangerous:

> Remember that you have a duty of care to yourself and other staff members as well as the patient – **do not take risks**.

> **Be safe** – do not see this man on your own; if you meet him in a room (rather than an open area) make sure that he is away from the door and that you are close to the door; and if you are wearing a tie, remove it.

The circumstances mean that it will clearly not be possible to get a reliable and useful medical history from the patient. Use any other sources of information that may be available, as described in Section 1.3.29, with points of particular importance being the speed of onset of symptoms; drug or alcohol ingestion/withdrawal; recent history of head trauma; associated symptoms including headache, seizures and vomiting; and a history of significant past or current medical illness.

Examination and investigation

As with history taking, it will not be possible to perform a physical examination and pursue investigation in the usual manner if the patient is not cooperative. Try to glean as much information as you can from:

> Inspection – are there any signs of trauma, particularly to the head? Are there any localising neurological signs, eg is the patient moving both arms in the same sort of way? Are there any other features that suggest significant medical illness, eg rash?

> Vital signs – if the patient will allow these to be checked: fever and/or hypotension are not features of psychiatric illness.

If possible, check finger-prick blood glucose. Other investigations will be determined by clinical suspicion and the willingness (or otherwise) of the patient to cooperate; urine toxicology maybe helpful.

Key point

Write notes that clearly describe the situation

Your notes in the medical record must give a clear and precise description of the situation. Do not use vague terms such as 'patient uncooperative'. What did they say? Write it down in quotes: patient said 'piss off…go away'. How did they appear – 'bleeding from head wound and agitated; shouting out loud, sweating, shaking and tremulous; and holding onto a chair and threatening to use it as a weapon'.

Management

If the patient is hypoglycaemic (blood glucose <2.5 mmol/L) try to encourage them to drink or eat something sweet, but do not give them a hot drink which they might spill over themselves or throw over you. Obtaining intravenous access is not likely to be straightforward: give glucagon 1 mg IM if parenteral treatment is required.

If the patient has another specific medical or surgical diagnosis, then this will require appropriate treatment, but before such treatment can be administered it will be necessary to have a practical strategy for dealing with violence or aggression.

De-escalation techniques

Try to keep calm. Introduce yourself and reassure the patient: speak clearly; do not shout; minimise eye contact; and always maintain a safe distance. Ask the patient what the problem is:

acknowledge their feelings and empathise as appropriate; try to establish an emotional relationship ('I'm trying to help'); and attempt to address any immediate problems or explain why you cannot do so.

Sedation

If the patient needs further assessment or treatment and is not calmed by discussion and de-escalation techniques then sedation may be required as a last resort. The synergistic use of an antipsychotic and a benzodiazepine is often recommended: the benzodiazepine reducing the dose of antipsychotic necessary to produce calm and therefore limiting the risk of oversedation and other side effects. The most desirable end point of using sedatives in the context of agitation is a calm and cooperative patient, not an unresponsive one – which is sometimes a difficult balance to achieve. Remember that patients with Parkinson's disease may have significant reactions to commonly used antipsychotics and may be better suited to a benzodiazepine-only strategy.

Hazard

Sedation of the violent or aggressive patient

The physician administering sedation must be confident in airway management, have appropriate backup from the ICU and must also have the correct doses of antagonists available.

Perform sedation as follows:

> Step 1 – begin by encouraging the patient to take oral sedation: the oral route being the safest but with the requirement for patient cooperation, and the downside that oral medications take some time to be absorbed. Try lorazepam 1–4 mg stat and haloperidol 2.5 mg stat (rising to 5–10 mg if needed).

> Step 2 – give intramuscular sedation, but be careful to avoid accidental needle-stick injury of individuals other than the patient and remember that the absorption profile of drugs given intramuscularly is also unpredictable. Try lorazepam 1–4 mg stat and haloperidol 2.5 mg stat (rising to 5–10 mg if needed).

> Step 3 – if the patient is *in extremis* and you think it essential to sedate them immediately: request four people trained in control and restraint (one for each arm and one for each leg); request an anaesthetist and ensure that resuscitation equipment is available; draw up several syringes, each containing a reasonable dose of intravenous benzodiazepine (eg lorazepam 4 mg); and when all are assembled restrain the patient, insert intravenous cannula, inject one syringe of benzodiazepine, wait 60 seconds and then repeat as necessary until sedation is achieved.

! Hazard

Do not take risks!
If you are confronted with a violent or aggressive patient and genuinely fear for your safety, keep yourself and others out of the patient's way until adequate help is available. If they are trying to leave the hospital then let them go, informing duty hospital manager and/or police as appropriate.

Key point

Where should the violent or aggressive patient be managed?

> If an underlying medical problem requiring admission for treatment is present – admit the patient to a medical ward when appropriate nursing supervision has been organised, eg one-to-one nurse in attendance.

> If the patient has a psychiatric disorder, but no medical disorder – it is up to a psychiatrist to decide if admission to a psychiatric unit is required. Medical admission is not recommended.

> If they have no underlying psychiatric or medical disorder – *the person should not remain in hospital*; the police should deal with any violent behaviour. It may be appropriate to call hospital security pending the arrival of the police.

Acute medicine: Section 2

2 Diseases and treatments

2.1 Overdoses

The general clinical approach to the patient who has taken an overdose is described in Section 1.3.33, to the patient who is in circulatory shock in Section 1.3.2 and to the patient in coma in Section 1.3.29.

Key point

For any patient who has taken an overdose seek advice sooner rather than later from Toxbase (www.toxbase.org – this website requires hospital registration to access the service) or by phoning the National Poisons Information Service (NPIS), who offer a 24-hour telephone information line. For contact details see their website (www.npis.org/).

2.1.1 Prevention of drug absorption from the gut

Activated charcoal

This is the preferred method of gut decontamination if the dose of toxin taken is likely to cause moderate to severe toxicity. The single dose (50 g for adults) can be given up to 1 hour after ingestion, but note that some drugs are not readily adsorbed to charcoal and that repeated doses may be useful for some toxins (Table 26).

Hazard

Charcoal is dangerous if aspirated.

Table 26   Use of activated charcoal after overdose

Toxins not absorbed by charcoal	Toxins for which repeated doses of charcoal may be useful
Iron salts Lithium Ethanol / methanol / ethylene glycol Acids/alkalis Organic solvents Mercury Lead Fluorides Potassium salts	Slow-release preparations Carbamazepine Dapsone Digoxin Paraquat Phenobarbitone Quinine Amanita phalloides (death cap mushroom)

Other techniques

Gastric lavage and/or emetics are now not used, studies having shown that they do not improve clinical outcome; they are definitely contraindicated in any patient who is unable to maintain their airway or following the ingestion of corrosives or organic solvents.

Whole bowel irrigation with polyethylene glycol solution, given orally or through a nasogastric tube until clear fluid appears per rectum, can be used following ingestion of slow-release preparations – lithium, iron, arsenic, lead oxide and zinc sulphate. However, it is contraindicated if there is an inability to maintain the airway and ileus, or if there is bowel obstruction or haemodynamic instability.

2.1.2 Management of overdoses of specific drugs

Paracetamol

Patients presenting with paracetamol overdose will usually have no symptoms related to paracetamol toxicity. Nausea and vomiting may occur, and right subcostal pain and tenderness suggest hepatic necrosis. The feared complication is acute liver failure, which may develop over days.

Key point

> The plasma paracetamol concentration should be checked in any patient suspected of having taken an overdose, at 4 hours post-ingestion (if they present earlier than the 4 hours).

> The decision about whether to immediately start N-acetylcysteine depends on how many hours after ingestion the patient presents; the amount of paracetamol ingested; and the results of any initial blood tests – always refer to Toxbase for the latest up-to-date advice.

> The treatment nomogram (Fig 42) can then be reviewed, in conjunction with the clinical history and blood tests, to decide whether N-acetylcysteine is required, or can be stopped (ie the level is below the treatment line).

> An accurate history is essential for the interpretation of the plasma paracetamol concentration (the nomogram is not reliable if the timing of the overdose is not clear). If there is any doubt then N-acetylcysteine should be given regardless of the level.

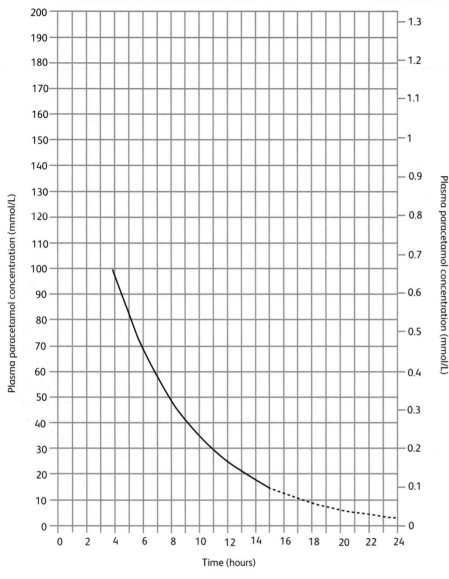

Fig 42 Paracetamol treatment lines. (Reproduced with permission from the Medicines and Healthcare products Regulatory Agency – contains public sector information licensed under the Open Government Licence v3.0.)

The dose of N-acetylcysteine for adults who weigh over 40 kg is 150 mg/kg in 200 mL 5% dextrose or 0.9% sodium chloride intravenously over 1 hour; then 50 mg/kg in 500 mL 5% dextrose or 0.9% sodium chloride over 4 hours; and then 100 mg/kg in 1,000 mL 5% dextrose or 0.9% sodium chloride over 16 hours. Continued N-acetylcysteine should be given at a rate of 150 mg/kg over 24 hours if the patient is symptomatic and/or there are abnormalities on investigation (raised prothrombin time (PT)/INR and/or elevated plasma creatinine and/or acidosis).

Anaphylactoid reactions to N-acetylcysteine occur in 20% of patients and include nausea, flushing, urticaria, angio-oedema, bronchospasm and hypotension. These usually occur early and often resolve if N-acetylcysteine is stopped. Intravenous chlorphenamine can then be given (and nebulised salbutamol, if bronchospasm is present), after which the infusion may be restarted at a lower rate.

Patients sometimes present with toxicologically trivial (but perhaps psychiatrically very significant) overdoses of paracetamol. As a rough guide, doses of less than 75 mg/kg in a 24-hour period are unlikely to be toxic, although repeated ingestion over 2 days or more will clearly increase this risk. Those who consume more than 150 mg/kg in any 24-hour period are at risk of serious toxicity.

Key point

Following paracetamol overdose specialist advice from a liver centre should be sought in the presence of *any* of the following indicators of severe hepatotoxicity:

> acidosis (pH <7.3), elevated lactate (>3.5 mmol/L) or hypotension (mean arterial pressure <60 mmHg) despite adequate fluid resuscitation

> INR is >2 at 24 hours post ingestion, >3 at 48 hours, or any rise in INR at 72 hours

> plasma creatinine is >200 µmol/L

> hypoglycaemia

> encephalopathy.

Tricyclic antidepressants

Coma, convulsions and arrhythmias are the most serious signs of toxicity. Tachycardia and QRS prolongation (>100 ms) on the ECG indicate severe poisoning. Anticholinergic effects include blurred vision, dry mouth, pupillary dilation and urinary retention. Central effects include confusion, drowsiness, nystagmus, ataxia, hyperreflexia and hyperthermia.

The most important aspects of management are cardiac monitoring and efforts to increase urinary excretion of the tricyclic by alkaline diuresis:

> Place on cardiac monitor – dysrhythmias may respond to correction of hypoxia and acidosis, but antiarrhythmic drugs may be necessary – although some can exacerbate the toxic effects of tricyclics (seek expert advice).

> Correct hypotension with fluid resuscitation with crystalloid fluid.

> Urinary alkalinisation with sodium bicarbonate is indicated if there is systemic acidosis, prolonged QRS, ventricular arrhythmias, hypotension resistant to fluids or cardiac arrest. Ensure adequate fluid resuscitation prior to considering infusion of 50–100 mL of 8.4% sodium bicarbonate, ideally via a central line (alternative concentrations of sodium bicarbonate can also be used). Further sodium bicarbonate can be given if required, targeting an arterial blood gas pH of 7.5.

> Give intravenous benzodiazepine for convulsions.

Salicylates

The important clinical features are hyperventilation, tinnitus, deafness, sweating, vasodilatation, convulsions, coma and death.

Important aspects of management are to check arterial blood gases (ABGs) – respiratory alkalosis and/or metabolic acidosis can be expected. If salicylate levels are >500 mg/L (3.6 mmol/L) then consider alkaline diuresis with sodium bicarbonate (see Toxbase for details); if they are >700 mg/L (5.1 mmol/L), consider haemodialysis.

3 Investigations and practical procedures

3.1 Central venous lines

3.1.1 Indications, contraindications, consent and preparation

Indications for insertion of a central line

These include the infusion of fluids (including parenteral feeding); the infusion of drugs, eg inotropes and hypertonic solutions; measurement of the central venous pressure (CVP); insertion of a temporary pacing wire, access for haemodialysis/haemofiltration or when peripheral access is difficult.

Contraindications to insertion of a central line

There are no absolute contraindications, but relative contraindications include: abnormal clotting, distorted/abnormal anatomy, localised infection at entry point, proximal vascular injury or an uncooperative patient. Severe respiratory disease and COPD are relative contraindications especially for the subclavian approach because a pneumothorax may precipitate respiratory failure; and local sepsis. If possible, correct marked hypovolaemia prior to central vein cannulation. This is because the technique is typically more difficult, time consuming and carries more risk of complications. Patients with a history of difficult cannulations should be supervised by an experienced physician.

Consent for insertion of a central line

Whether or not verbal or written consent for central line insertion should be obtained from the patient will depend on the clinical context. If central lines are being inserted in the non-emergency situation then written consent (either from the patient or relative, depending on situation) will be required in most hospitals, and many will have specific consent forms for the purpose. The broad principles of informed consent apply: patients need to know and understand the indication for the procedure, the details of the procedure – including the need to lie still and (relatively) flat; and the potential complications (Table 27).

Preparation for central line insertion

> Check platelet count and clotting.

> Obtain informed consent.

> Ensure adequate monitoring is available – cardiac monitor and pulse oximeter.

> Prepare equipment:

> > Dressing pack, drapes and gloves (all sterile).

> > Local anaesthetic, syringe and needle.

> Seldinger catheter set with 5 mL syringe, introducer needle, guidewire, dilator and central line, or a 16 G long cannula.

> Prepare ultrasound machine with transducer, sterile probe cover, sterile gel

> Saline or Hepsal flush.

> Three-way tap (×3 if triple lumen catheter).

> Small scalpel blade, silk suture and sterile occlusive dressing.

Key point

Technique for central line insertion
Unless it is an emergency and/or ultrasound is not available, then all central venous catheters should be inserted under direct ultrasound guidance.

Table 27	Complications arising from central line insertion	
Frequency	**Internal jugular**	**Subclavian**
Common	Arterial puncture (2–8%) Pneumothorax (<1%) Bleeding / bruising / haematoma formation Infection	Arterial puncture (2–4%) Pneumothorax/haemopneumothorax (1–2.5%) Bleeding / bruising / haematoma formation Infection
Less common/rare	Nerve damage Arteriovenous fistula Venous thrombosis Lost catheters	Nerve damage Chylothorax (especially left-sided lines) Arteriovenous fistula Venous thrombosis Lost catheters

It is not sensible to inform a patient of every possible complication that might arise from central line insertion (or any other procedure), but – in the context of explaining the indications and potential benefits to them of the procedure – it would be expected that they would be told of the common problems that can arise.

3.1.2 Specific techniques for insertion of central lines

Ultrasound-guided internal jugular vein cannulation using the Seldinger technique

> Lie the patient down, preferably with a head-down tilt, and turn their head away from the side you intend to cannulate.

> Identify your landmarks (Fig 43) – the internal jugular vein lies superficial, lateral and parallel to the carotid artery. Identify the apex of the triangle formed by the two heads of the sternocleidomastoid muscle at the level of the thyroid cartilage. A 'high approach' minimises the risk of pneumothorax.

> Apply gel and pre-scan the neck with the ultrasound – keep the probe in the short axis and perpendicular to the skin.

> Orientate yourself and identify your landmarks and vessels as described above. Make sure you clearly differentiate the vein from the artery – the internal jugular vein is typically much larger than the artery, is compressible, has a thinner wall and will increase in diameter with the Valsalva manoeuver or intra-abdominal pressure. Colour Doppler can also be used if necessary. Only when completely happy, proceed with the following steps.

> Gown and glove, clean and drape the skin.

> Flush the lumen(s) of the central line with saline or Hepsal and ensure you have all your equipment within easy reach.

> Put sterile gel on the transducer, cover with sterile probe cover and fix with elastic bands. Leave in safe place when not in use.

> Reorientate anatomy using the ultrasound then infiltrate the skin and subcutaneous tissue with 1% lidocaine.

> Attach the introducer needle to the 5 or 10 mL syringe and draw up 1 mL saline. Ensure the transducer is perpendicular to the vessel and insert the needle in the midline of the transducer.

> Slowly advance using a jackhammer technique, making sure you visualise the needle on the ultrasound image and aspirating as you go.

> Observe the needle entering the vessel wall with associated flashback of blood.

> Once you are in the vein and can aspirate blood freely, remove the syringe and occlude the end of the needle with your finger to prevent air embolism.

> Pass the guidewire into the vein, ensuring that it passes freely – remove the wire if there is any resistance and check that blood can still be aspirated easily, then try again.

> Remove the needle, leaving the wire in the vein.

> Observe the guidewire in the vein using the ultrasound.

> Nick the skin at the base of the wire with the small scalpel blade to allow easy passage of the dilator – if there is resistance do not use force, which can crimp the guidewire or the end of the dilator. The usual explanation is that an adequate nick has not been made with the scalpel blade.

> Pass the dilator over the wire through the subcutaneous tissue using a twisting motion and then remove it, leaving the wire *in situ*.

> Pass the central line over the wire into the vein. Keep hold of the wire at all times.

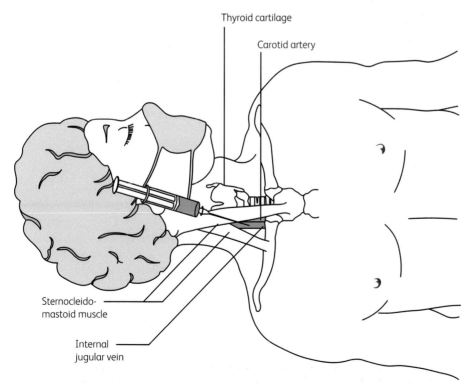

Thyroid cartilage

Carotid artery

Sternocleido-mastoid muscle

Internal jugular vein

Fig 43 Cannulation of the internal jugular vein.

- Remove the wire and check that you can aspirate blood freely through all ports – confirm venous placement either using blood gas analyser or transduce the line.

- With the line in place, flush with saline and close the line off to air.

- Secure with sutures, clean then place a sterile occlusive dressing over the site.

- Confirm position with chest X-ray.

If measurement of the CVP is needed, attach the manometer set to the patient and adjust the zero reference point on the manometer so it is at the level of the patient's right atrium (midaxillary line). Alternatively, an electronic transducer and oscilloscope may be used to continuously measure the CVP, which also need to be zeroed and calibrated prior to use.

Ultrasound-guided femoral vein cannulation using the Seldinger technique

- Position the patient as flat as possible in the supine position with the hip abducted and externally rotated, and knee slightly flexed.

- Apply gel and pre-scan the groin with the ultrasound – keep the probe in the short axis and perpendicular to the skin.

- Identify your landmarks (Fig 44) – the femoral vein lies directly medial to the femoral artery in the femoral triangle (nerve, artery, vein and 'Y-fronts' (NAVY)).

- Using the ultrasound as your guide, the needle needs to be inserted at an angle of 20–30° and aimed cephalad.

- Follow remainder of points as described above.

Vein ———

Artery ———

Nerve ———

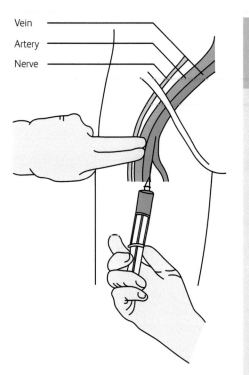

Fig 44 Cannulation of the femoral vein.

Ultrasound-guided subclavian vein cannulation using the Seldinger technique

- Position the patient with a head-down tilt and turn the head away from the side you wish to cannulate.

- Note that interference from the clavicle complicates the use of ultrasound in cannulating the subclavian vein and as such, the landmark technique is still in use for this procedure. However, the ultrasound guided infraclavicular technique allows cannulation of the subclavian or proximal axillary vein.

- Identify your landmarks – the clavicle, pleural lines as well as the artery and vein should be clearly identified below the distal half of the clavicle.

- The needle needs to be inserted just below the lower border of the clavicle, making sure it is kept in the horizontal plane and directed medially.

- Follow remainder of points described above.

! Hazard

Do not make a bad situation worse:

- If the carotid artery is punctured and a haematoma forms, do not attempt internal jugular vein cannulation on the other side (especially in patients with abnormal clotting) – bilateral haematomas may result in airway compromise; seek experienced help – cannulation of the subclavian or femoral vein are most likely to be appropriate.

- Do not attempt to cannulate the opposite subclavian vessel if the first attempt was unsuccessful – giving a patient bilateral pneumothoraces can be fatal; do a check chest radiograph or cannulate the internal jugular or femoral vein instead.

- In ventilated patients even a small pneumothorax must be treated with a chest drain as it may rapidly turn into a tension pneumothorax.

3.1.3 Interpretation of central venous pressure measurements

 Key point

Before measuring the central venous pressure (CVP) ensure that the system has been zeroed to the midaxillary reference point and that the venous pressure swings with respiration.

The CVP gives an indication of the patient's blood volume but is also affected by the contractile state of the myocardium, venous tone, intrathoracic pressure and pulmonary arterial pressure. It does not always provide accurate information on left-sided

Table 28	Causes of an abnormal CVP	
CVP reading	Real or artefact?	Cause
High	Genuine	Fluid overload Right ventricular failure, eg right ventricular infarction Massive PE Cardiac tamponade Tension pneumothorax
	Error	Incorrect zero Incorrect placement – catheter tip in right ventricle will give an unexpectedly high pressure Blocked catheter – causes a sustained high reading with a damped waveform Infusion of fluid, eg through an infusion pump, at the same time the pressure is being measured
Low	Genuine	Hypovolaemia Septic shock Anaphylactic shock
	Error	Incorrect zero

CVP, central venous pressure; PE, pulmonary embolism.

cardiac filling pressures, which can be low even though the CVP is normal or high, the classic example of this being severe pulmonary embolism (PE).

The normal range for the CVP is +3 cm to +8 cm if zero is defined as 5 cm below the angle of Louis (sometimes incorrectly called the 'method of Louis') or +7 cm to +12 cm if zero is defined according to the phlebostatic axis (the midpoint between the anterior and posterior surfaces of the chest at the level of the fourth intercostal space). Causes of an abnormal CVP are shown in Table 28.

3.2 Lumbar puncture

Indications for performing a lumbar puncture

Diagnostic indications are meningitis, encephalitis, subarachnoid haemorrhage (SAH) and intrathecal malignancy.

Therapeutic indications are intrathecal drug administration and benign intracranial hypertension.

Contraindications to performing a lumbar puncture

These include raised intracranial pressure; posterior fossa or spinal cord mass lesions; local sepsis; and a bleeding tendency.

Key point

Lumbar puncture and risk of coning
If a patient is unconscious, drowsy or has clinical features of raised intracranial pressure or focal neurological signs, then a CT scan must be performed prior to lumbar puncture. Antibiotic treatment should be started immediately if there is likely to be a delay and meningitis is a diagnostic possibility.

Preparation

> Check platelet count and clotting.

> Obtain informed consent.

> Prepare equipment:

> dressing pack, gown, drapes and gloves (all sterile)

> local anaesthetic, syringe and needles

> antiseptic

> lumbar puncture needles and sterile manometer

> sample tubes (serum glucose bottle, and three sterile 20 mL containers for: differential counts / cytology; microscopy, culture and sensitivity (M/C/S); and viral polymerase chain reaction (PCR) and protein estimation, and a fourth sterile container protected from light for xanthochromia if performed separately from cell count locally).

Technique

> Ask the patient to lie on the bed (Fig 45a) – positioning is all-important; the knees should be drawn up towards the chest to open the space between the spinous processes, and the spine should be parallel to the bed. It may help to place a pillow between legs.

> Gown and glove up.

> Prepare the skin with antiseptic and cover with sterile drapes – remember to cover top of hip to allow checking of anatomical landmarks.

> Locate the puncture site (L3/L4 or L4/L5).

> Anaesthetise the skin and subcutaneous tissues with 5–10 mL 1% lidocaine (lignocaine) using a 25 G needle; then switch to an 18 G needle and infiltrate the deeper tissues.

> Assemble the manometer and unscrew the tops of the sterile containers.

> Insert the lumbar puncture needle at 90° to the skin – advance slowly, aiming between two spinous processes and slightly towards

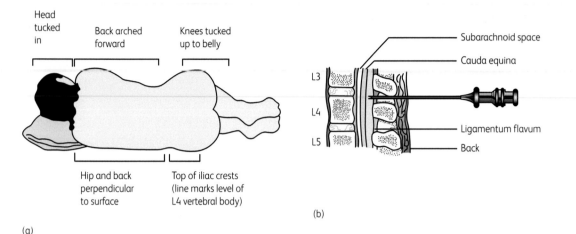

Head tucked in
Back arched forward
Knees tucked up to belly

Hip and back perpendicular to surface
Top of iliac crests (line marks level of L4 vertebral body)

(a)

Subarachnoid space
Cauda equina
L3
L4
Ligamentum flavum
L5
Back

(b)

Fig 45 Technique for lumbar puncture. **(a)** The patient should be curled up to increase the space between the vertebrae; **(b)** the needle should be advanced slowly until it penetrates the ligamentum flavum – a flashback of CSF when the stylet is removed indicates correct positioning.

umbilicus. There is a slight loss of resistance as the needle enters the dural space (Fig 45b).

> Remove the stylet and ensure that cerebrospinal fluid (CSF) drips freely from the needle – if no CSF is forthcoming, insert the stylet and advance the needle a few millimetres and check again.

> Attach the manometer and measure the pressure (normal 6–15 cm water).

> Collect CSF samples:

> 5 drops for biochemistry, may need separate xanthochromia sample, depending on policy.

> 10 drops for bacteriology (ask for urgent microscopy and Gram stain, and culture, sensitivities and viral studies).

> 10 drops for cytology.

> Remove the needle and dress the wound.

> Ask the patient to remain lying flat for 2–4 hours to reduce the severity of post-lumbar puncture headache and to remain well hydrated.

Always send blood samples for glucose and protein estimation at the same time as CSF samples: the CSF glucose concentration is normally 60–80% of the blood level. In cases of suspected subarachnoid haemorrhage (SAH) the red cell count in consecutive samples can help to distinguish SAH from a bloody tap, and the samples should also be examined for xanthochromia (oxyhaemoglobin and bilirubin).

Normal values and values in disease for CSF pressure, cell counts, glucose concentration and protein concentration are shown in Table 29.

3.3 Cardiac pacing

There are three common types of cardiac pacing – transvenous endocardial (may be temporary or permanent), epicardial (in association with cardiac surgery) and transcutaneous/external.

Common indications for pacing
Bradyarrhythmias

> Temporary pacing:

> The decision to pace is based on the presence of haemodynamic compromise or potential to do so rather than the specific rhythm.

> Patients with second- or third-degree atrioventricular (AV) block may need temporary pacing prior to general anaesthesia.

Table 29 Cerebrospinal fluid findings in various conditions				
	Pressure (cmH$_2$O)	White cells (per µL)	Protein (g/L)	Glucose (mmol/L)
Normal	6–15	≤5 mononuclear cells	0.2–0.4	2.5–4.5
Bacterial meningitis	Normal or ↑	↑↑↑ polymorphs	1–5	0.2–2.2
Viral meningitis	Normal or ↑	↑ to ↑↑ lymphocytes	≤1	Normal
Tumour	Normal or ↑	0–100s mononuclear cells Malignant cells also possible	↑↑	Normal or ↓

Medical Masterclass Third edition

> Patients with second- or third-degree heart block in association with an acute myocardial infarction may require pacing (this may be complicated by the need to obtain central venous access in someone who has received thrombolysis).

> Permanent pacing:

> Class-1 indications are chronic, symptomatic second- or third-degree AV block, and sinoatrial node dysfunction with recurrent syncope.

> Class-2 indications are asymptomatic third-degree AV block and resistant sinus bradycardia.

Tachyarrhythmias

Some tachyarrhythmias (AV nodal re-entrant tachycardia, AV re-entry tachycardia, atrial flutter and VT) may be treated by pacing or by premature electrical stimulation: this may be done by a temporary transvenous pacing wire or – if persistent – by a permanent system.

Technique for external pacing

After explaining to the patient what you are going to do ensure they have adequate sedation and analgesia:

> Place one electrode in a position equivalent to lead V2–V3 of the ECG, with the other either over the apex of the heart or on the posterior of the chest below the left scapula (Fig 46)

> Set the pacing box to demand, with a rate of approximately 60 beats per minute.

> Connect the leads to the patient and slowly increase the current; 50–100 mA is usually required.

> Ventricular capture is indicated when a pacing spike is associated with a ventricular complex and a palpable pulse wave.

> Make immediate arrangements for transvenous pacing – external pacing is unreliable and should be continued for as short a period as possible.

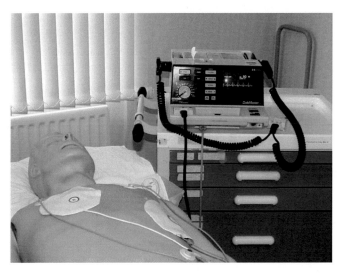

Fig 46 External pacing with a modern monitor/defibrillator/external pacer.

If external pacing is unsuccessful ensure there is adequate current, then try other electrodes or electrode positions, percussion pacing (forceful, rhythmic thumping of the left anterior chest), isoprenaline infusion or immediate transvenous pacing.

Common problems of transvenous pacing

The procedure for temporary transvenous pacing is beyond the scope of this book, but it is important for all doctors working on hospital wards to be aware of the common problems that can arise with

transvenous pacing once it has been established:

> Increasing threshold – temporary transvenous pacemakers should have their threshold tested at least daily as this often increases over time. Testing is done by gradually turning down the pacemaker current until failure to capture occurs. The pacemaker output should be set at three times the threshold voltage or 3 volts, whichever is the higher. Increasing threshold is an indication for repositioning of the wire or urgent permanent pacing (Fig 47).

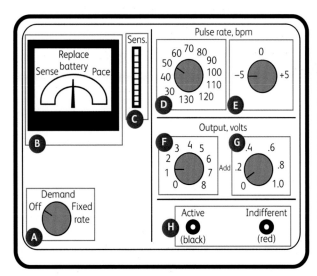

A Mode: demand vs fixed
B Pointer: allows you to see whether an intrinsic beat is sensed or if the patient is being paced
C Sensitivity should be set at 1.0
D Rate setting
E Rate adjustment by ±5 bpm
F & G Voltage adjustment: should be set at 3 volts above threshold
H Lead terminals

Fig 47 A common type of pacemaker generator.

- Loss of electrical continuity – the commonest reason for sudden failure of a pacemaker to work, which may result in symptomatic bradycardia, is a loose connection. There are generally four connections between the pacing electrodes and the pacemaker box: check them all.

- Electrode displacement – the tip of the transvenous pacemaker should be in the right ventricle; migration of the pacing wire can lead to an increasing threshold or sudden bradycardia.

Key point

If a temporary pacemaker suddenly stops working, always check the connections before you do anything else.

3.4 Elective direct-current cardioversion

Indication and preparation

The indication for elective DC cardioversion is tachyarrhythmias causing cardiovascular compromise, significant symptoms or symptoms that are resistant to drug therapy.

Consider anticoagulation – cardioversion of atrial fibrillation (AF) has a thromboembolic risk of around 5%, hence patients should be therapeutically anticoagulated for 6 weeks before elective cardioversion for this indication.

Check the electrolytes and ensure that digoxin toxicity has been excluded.

Technique

The patient should be starved in case of the need for intubation.

- Obtain informed consent.

- Give oxygen by facemask.

- Ensure there is adequate intravenous access.

- Ensure there is adequate monitoring and that a defibrillator is available – ECG electrodes must be applied to the chest and connected to the defibrillator.

- Ensure the availability of emergency drugs.

- Ensure there is adequate sedation/analgesia – experienced personnel may perform elective cardioversion under sedation alone; many prefer general anaesthesia.

- Apply gel pads to position V2–V3 on the anterior chest and over the apex of the heart.

- Ensure the defibrillator is set to apply an (R-wave) synchronised shock.

- Charge the defibrillator while the paddles are applied to the patient's chest; appropriate starting voltages depend on the arrhythmia: AF or broad complex tachycardia – 120–150 J biphasic; atrial flutter / supraventricular tachycardia (SVT) – 70–120 J biphasic.

- Discharge the current only after ensuring that it is safe to do so. Discharging during maximum expiration reduces impedance and may improve likelihood of success.

- Recheck the cardiac rhythm and the patient's observations.

- If unsuccessful, increase energy in increments as per local policy.

3.5 Intercostal chest drain insertion

Indications

- Pneumothorax:

  - In any ventilated patient.

  - Tension pneumothorax after initial needle thoracocentesis.

  - Persistent or recurrent pneumothorax after simple aspiration.

  - Large secondary spontaneous pneumothorax in patients aged over 50 years.

- Malignant pleural effusion.

- Empyema and complicated parapneumonic pleural effusion.

- Traumatic haemopneumothorax.

- Postoperative, eg thoracotomy, oesophagectomy and cardiac surgery.

Small-bore chest drains (10–14 Fr) are recommended: they are as effective as large-bore tubes in most circumstances and are better tolerated by the patient. Large-bore tubes (28–32 Fr) should be used for haemothoraces and in the event of failure to drain a pneumothorax via a small-bore tube: they may also still have a role in the treatment of empyema, although increasing success is being seen with small-bore drains in conjunction with thrombolytic therapy.

It is strongly recommended that all chest drains for fluid are inserted under ultrasound guidance and this requires specialist training. Ultrasound is of limited use in the context of a pneumothorax given the poor transmission of sound waves through air.

Hazard

Tension pneumothorax Never wait for a chest radiograph if a tension pneumothorax has been diagnosed on clinical grounds – do an immediate needle thoracocentesis and then insert a chest drain.

Preparation

Hazard

Begin by careful radiological assessment – you do not want to insert a drain into an emphysematous bulla by mistake.

> Risk assessment – coagulopathy or platelet deficit should be corrected prior to chest drain insertion. If the patient is on warfarin this should be stopped, with the aim of an INR <1.5 prior to the procedure.

> Explain the benefits, risks and technique of the procedure and obtain written consent from the patient, unless in an emergency situation.

> Intravenous access – this should be established in all patients. If the procedure is being done for a haemothorax make sure that you have two large-bore intravenous cannulae in place and blood available for transfusion before starting the procedure.

> Monitoring – the patient should be on oxygen during the procedure, with the monitoring of oxygen saturations throughout.

> Pre-medication – this should be considered and offered to every patient who is not *in extremis*, eg midazolam (1–5 mg IV).

> Equipment – make sure you have everything you need on the trolley before you start: basic sterile pack; local anaesthetic and syringes with orange and green needles; chest drain insertion pack (Fig 48) complete with chest drain (and connectors), guide wire and dilators (replaced by Spencer Wells forceps if it is a large-bore drain), scalpel and handle, syringe and needle; scissors; suture 1/0 or 2/0 silk; dressings; and an underwater seal bottle with connections.

Technique

> Position the patient – ideally in a semi-recumbent position with their hand resting behind their head.

> Identify the landmarks (Fig 49) – the safest position for chest drain insertion is in the fifth intercostal space in the midaxillary line. In a patient without large breasts this will

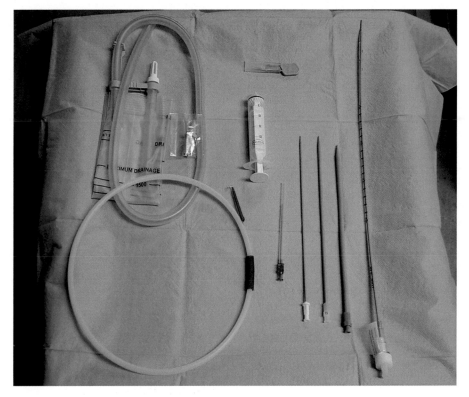

Fig 48 Chest drain insertion pack.

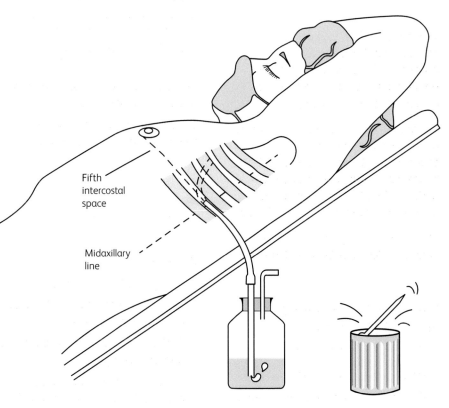

Fifth intercostal space

Midaxillary line

Fig 49 Landmarks for insertion of an intercostal chest drain.

be at the level of the nipple; in someone with large breasts select the intercostal space a hand's width below the axilla.

> Clean and drape the skin – aseptic technique should be observed at all times.

> Infiltrate the skin with local anaesthetic using the orange needle and then infiltrate down to the pleura using the green needle – then go through the pleura to aspirate air or fluid.

Hazard

A chest drain should not be inserted if free air or fluid cannot be aspirated with a needle at the time of introduction of local anaesthesia – get further image guidance.

Small-bore chest drain insertion using a Seldinger technique

> Insert the supplied needle into the pleural space, ensuring you aspirate to reconfirm position.

> Pass the guidewire through the needle and then carefully withdraw the needle leaving the guidewire *in situ*.

> Pass the dilator over the guidewire and through the subcutaneous tissue into the pleural space. A small incision in the skin and subcutaneous tissue may be necessary prior to dilator insertion. Withdraw the dilator, leaving the guidewire *in situ*.

> Pass the chest drain over the guidewire into the pleural space and then withdraw the guidewire.

> Connect the chest drain to an underwater seal and confirm position – oscillation, fluid drainage and bubbling.

> Secure the drain in place with a 1/0 or 2/0 silk suture – tie it so that the skin is closed either side of the drain and then wrap it around and tie

it to the drain as many times as its length allows.

> Apply a clear, impervious dressing and ensure the joins between drain and connectors are secured.

Hazard

You must keep hold of the guidewire at all times when inserting a small-bore chest drain using the Seldinger technique!

Large-bore chest drain insertion

> Make a 2–3 cm incision through the skin and subcutaneous adipose tissue along the line of the intercostal space, just above the edge of the lower rib.

> Bluntly dissect down to the pleura using forceps.

> Puncture the parietal pleura with the tip of the forceps and then insert your finger to enlarge the hole. Sweep your finger around to clear any adhesions or clots. Make sure there is adequate space to insert the drain without using force.

> Remove any trochar from the chest drain and slide the drain over your finger into the thoracic cavity.

> Connect the chest drain to an underwater seal and confirm position – oscillation, fluid drainage and bubbling.

> Secure the drain in place with a 1/0 or 2/0 silk suture – tie it so that the skin is closed either side of the drain and then wrap it around and tie it to the drain as many times as its length allows.

> Apply a clear, impervious dressing and ensure the joins between drain and connectors are secured.

After the procedure

Observe that the drain is functioning – oscillation with respiration, fluid drainage and/or bubbling. Order a chest radiograph

to confirm correct positioning of the drain. Prescribe adequate analgesia.

Inform nursing staff of requirements for managing the chest drain:

> Never clamp a bubbling chest drain.

> Controlled drainage of a large pleural effusion to prevent re-expansion pulmonary oedema.

> Accurate recording of fluid drainage and daily function of the chest drain.

Daily assessment of the patient and review of the chest drain is vital. A repeat chest radiograph should be obtained if fluid stops draining, bubbling stops, there is no clear evidence of oscillation of the chest drain or there are concerns with the patient's condition. However, it is not necessary to repeat the chest radiograph daily as a routine.

The chest drain can be removed if there is no fluid drainage or bubbling for >24 hours following radiographic confirmation of resolution of the effusion or pneumothorax. In malignant effusions pleurodesis may be considered prior to removal. The chest radiograph should be repeated following removal of the drain.

Key point

If there is a failure of the fluid level to swing with respiration, check:

> Is the tube kinked?

> Is the tube blocked?

> Is the tube in the wrong position?

Key point

Causes of a persistent pneumothorax:
> large primary leak

> leakage at the skin or underwater seal

> bronchopleural fistula.

Complications of inserting a chest drain

> Damage to intrathoracic and/or abdominal organs or vessels – these can be avoided by using the finger sweep and never using the trochar for large-bore chest drain insertion.

> Damage to the intercostal nerve, artery or vein – avoid making the incision below the rib as the intercostal nerves and vessels lie beneath the lower edge of the rib.

> Sepsis: empyema formation or cellulitis – ensure complete aseptic technique, and do not leave chest drains in for longer than necessary.

> Pulmonary oedema if the lung expands rapidly following drainage of a large pleural effusion – drainage of pleural fluid should be limited to around 200 mL/h.

> Surgical emphysema.

> Haematoma – check that there are no clotting or platelet abnormalities prior to insertion.

> Pain – ensure there is adequate analgesia.

3.6 Arterial blood gases

3.6.1 Measurement of arterial blood gases

Indications for arterial blood gases (ABGs) include pulse oximetry showing PO_2 <92% and any acute unexplained severe illness. There are no absolute contraindications, although severe bleeding disorder is a relative contraindication.

Explain the procedure to the patient – those who have had ABGs performed know how painful they can be – and then proceed as follows.

Preparation

> Site – choose the site for arterial puncture carefully: radial, brachial or femoral. The radial is most commonly used, in which case first perform the Allen test to check the patency of the ulnar artery: ask the patient to clench their fist firmly, applying pressure to the radial artery, and then asking them to relax their fist, at which point the hand should pink up within 10 seconds.

> Equipment – before taking the sample, ensure that you know where the blood gas machine is and how to use it! Assemble alcohol swabs and a preheparinised ABG syringe or a 2 mL syringe into which you have drawn up and then expelled 0.5 mL 5,000 U/mL heparin through an appropriate needle: 25 G needles are perfectly adequate to obtain ABG samples from a radial artery; 18 G or 23 G are needed for a femoral sample.

Technique

> After gloving up, lay the index and middle fingers of your non-dominant hand along the line of the artery as a guide (Fig 50).

> For radial and brachial samples hold the syringe at 45–60° to the skin and slowly advance in the line of the artery; for femoral samples hold the syringe at 90° to the skin. There is debate over the use of lidocaine (lignocaine): while this is undoubtedly useful at easing pain if you are unlucky enough to fail first time, its use is painful in itself and it often makes palpation of the artery more difficult.

> A flush of blood indicates puncture of a vessel – with some ABG syringes, the arterial pressure will fill the syringe to a predetermined volume; in others you will need to aspirate 1–2 mL.

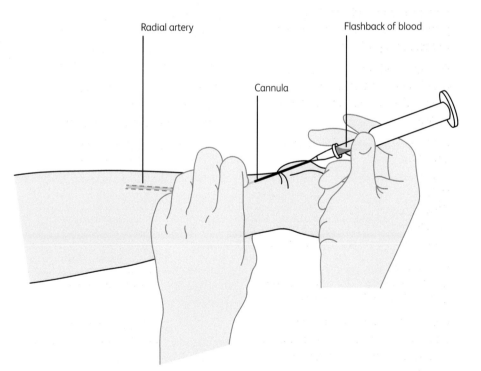

Fig 50 Taking a sample from the radial artery. The artery should be palpated with two fingers placed along the line of the artery. The needle should be inserted at 45–60° to the skin and slowly advanced in the direction of the artery. A flashback of blood indicates successful puncture.

- Apply pressure to the puncture site for 3 minutes (5 minutes if the patient is anticoagulated).
- Expel all air from the syringe; remove and dispose of the needle and cap the syringe.
- If there is to be a delay in processing the sample, pack it in ice.
- After the procedure check that bleeding has stopped, the main complication being haematoma.

3.6.2 Interpretation of arterial blood gases

Table 30 shows normal arterial blood gas (ABG) values.

The standard base excess (SBE) is a figure calculated by many blood gas machines as an aid to interpretation of ABG results. The principles of the calculation are as follows:

- Predict the pH that would arise in normal blood in the presence of the PCO_2 actually measured: if the PCO_2 is high, then the predicted pH is low; if the PCO_2 is low, then the predicted pH is high.
- Calculate the amount of acid or base that would have to be added to the blood to change the calculated pH into the pH as actually measured.
- This value is the base deficit or excess, in mmol/L, which quantifies the metabolic component of acid–base disturbance – the more negative the value of the SBE, the greater the degree of metabolic acidosis.

The types of metabolic and respiratory acid/base disturbances and their common causes are shown in Table 31.

Table 30 Normal ABG values

ABG	Normal range
pH	7.35–7.45
PCO_2	4.5–6.0 kPa
HCO_3	22–28 mmol/L
SBE	+ or –2 mmol/L
PO_2	10.5–14 kPa (breathing air)
O_2 saturation	95–100%

ABG, arterial blood gas; SBE, standard base excess.

Table 31 The types of metabolic and respiratory acid/base disturbances

Type of disturbance	pH	PCO₂	HCO₃	Base excess	Common causes
Metabolic acidosis	Low, or normal if there is respiratory compensation	Low due to a secondary respiratory alkalosis	Low – this is the primary abnormality in metabolic acidosis	Negative – this is the base deficit which quantifies the metabolic component of acid–base disturbances. The more negative the value, the greater the degree of metabolic acidosis	Lactic acidosis – exercise, shock and drugs (metformin) Ketoacidosis – diabetes Hyperchloraemic – bicarbonate wasting, eg renal losses and gastrointestinal fistulae High anion gap – poisoning, eg methanol and antifreeze
Respiratory acidosis	Low, or normal if there has been metabolic compensation	High – the primary abnormality is alveolar hypoventilation	Normal in an acute respiratory acidosis; high if there has been time for renal compensation	Normal	Acute – bronchopneumonia and severe acute asthma Chronic – COPD, neuromuscular disorders and restrictive lung diseases
Respiratory alkalosis	Elevated if acute, normal if there has been metabolic compensation	Low – the primary abnormality is alveolar hyperventilation	Normal in an acute respiratory alkalosis; low if there has been time for renal compensation	Normal	Anxiety Pain Hypoxia causing stimulation of the respiratory centre, eg pulmonary oedema and pneumonia Salicylate overdose – initially causes direct stimulation of the respiratory centre (but also uncouples oxidative phosphorylation leading to metabolic acidosis)
Metabolic alkalosis	Elevated – there is rarely significant respiratory compensation	Usually normal – little, if any, compensatory rise	Elevated – this is the primary abnormality in metabolic alkalosis	Positive – the more positive the value, the greater the degree of metabolic alkalosis	Chronic potassium depletion, eg vomiting and diuretics Chloride loss, eg vomiting

COPD, chronic obstructive pulmonary disease.

3.7 Airway management

Stridor, gurgling and snoring all suggest an airway at risk. Recognition of airway compromise depends on the following basic and lifesaving techniques – look, listen and feel:

> look for chest movement
> listen and feel for air movement at the nose and mouth.

All unconscious patients are at risk:

> A patient with a GCS score of <8 will need endotracheal intubation unless a cause can be rapidly found and corrected.
> Patients with a GCS score of 8–12 may need basic adjuncts to maintain airway patency.

Key point

Airway compromise results in rapid hypoxia and secondary brain injury. Airway management is the first priority in basic life support (BLS) (airway, breathing and circulation (ABC)) – but be wary of patients who are spontaneously ventilating but who cannot protect their airway because of a reduction in conscious level.

Key point

Oxygen should be given to all patients with decreased conscious levels unless specifically contraindicated.

3.7.1 Basic airway management

Opening the airway

Head tilt / chin lift

Loss of muscle control leads to occlusion of the airway by the tongue, epiglottis and soft palate. With the patient supine, extend the head on the neck by placing one hand on the forehead and pushing backwards. Place the fingers of the other hand under the tip of the jaw and lift the chin upwards (Fig 51a).

Jaw thrust

Place the fingers of both hands behind the angles of the mandible. Use upward pressure to lift the jaw forward (Fig 51b).

Hazard

Maintaining an airway in a patient with a suspected neck injury

The jaw thrust method is preferred because it results in less neck movement – but remember that patients with a neck injury are more likely to die from airway obstruction than damage due to neck movement.

Removing obstructions from the oropharynx

Solid foreign material should be removed using Magill forceps or a finger sweep under direct vision. Semisolid material or liquid should be removed using a Yankauer sucker.

Basic adjuncts to airway control

Oropharyngeal and nasopharyngeal airways help to prevent occlusion of the pharynx by the tongue and soft tissues (Fig 52). Patients with preserved laryngeal reflexes will generally not tolerate an oropharyngcal airway but may tolerate a nasopharyngeal one.

Insertion of an oropharyngeal airway

Select an airway that corresponds in length to the distance between the corner of the patient's mouth and the angle of the jaw. Open the patient's mouth. Introduce the airway upside down and rotate it 180° as it passes into the oropharynx. Reassess the airway.

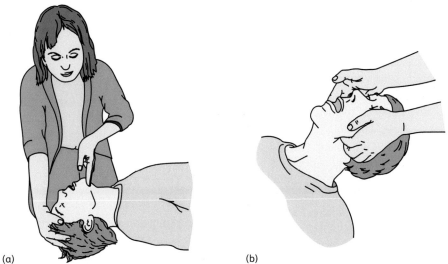

(a)   (b)

Fig 51 Opening the airway. **(a)** Head tilt / chin lift method: place one hand on the patient's forehead and the other under the point of the patient's chin, then tilt the head back to open the airway. **(b)** Jaw thrust method: with the index and middle fingers behind the angle of the mandible, apply upward and forward pressure to lift the jaw.

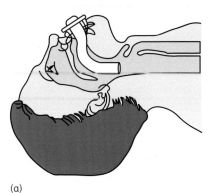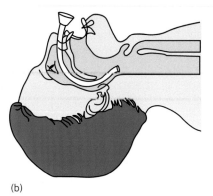

(a)   (b)

Fig 52 Basic adjuncts to airway control. **(a)** Oropharyngeal airway *in situ*.
(b) Nasopharyngeal airway *in situ*.

Hazard

Potential problems
with oropharyngeal
airways are:

> Incorrect insertion of the airway
can exacerbate the problem by
pushing the tongue further back.

> In the presence of laryngeal
reflexes, insertion of an
oropharyngeal airway can trigger
vomiting and laryngospasm.

Insertion of a nasopharyngeal airway

Select an airway with an external
diameter similar to the patient's little
finger. Place a safety pin through the
external flange of the airway to prevent it
being inhaled. Lubricate the airway. Check
the patency of the patient's nostrils and
for the presence of septal deviation – use
the nostril that seems easiest! Insert the
airway perpendicularly to the nostril,
along the floor of the nose. The airway
should pass easily, such that the flange
comes to rest at the nostril – if it does
not, remove it and try the other nostril.
Reassess the airway.

Hazard

Do not insert a
nasopharyngeal airway
if you suspect the
patient may have a basal skull fracture.

Key point

Ventilatory support
If the patient has
inadequate (or absent)
ventilation, then they require
ventilatory support. This can be
provided by mouth-to-mouth,
mouth-to-mask or bag-valve-mask
ventilation (the latter is a two-person
technique unless you are experienced)
while awaiting help. It is more
important to ventilate the patient
than for the inexperienced to attempt
intubation. Get help!

3.7.2 Tracheostomy

Indications

There are two main indications for
placement of a tracheostomy:

> Protection of the airway – following
surgery to the head or neck; trauma
or obstruction to the upper airway,
eg smoke inhalation or facial burns;
and bulbar or pseudobulbar palsies, to
prevent aspiration and to facilitate
the clearance of secretions.

> Reduction in work of breathing – a
tracheostomy can facilitate gradual
reduction in ventilatory support when
weaning from ventilation. This is
sometimes required in patients with
COPD or neuromuscular disorders.

Types of tracheostomy

Percutaneous tracheostomy

Seldinger technique and serial dilation
are used to insert tracheostomy.
This is usually done on ICU and can
be done under visualisation using a
bronchoscope. A track becomes
established about 10 days after
placement, at which point the
temporary tracheostomy should be
changed to one with a removable inner
tube to facilitate cleaning.

Hazard

If a percutaneous
tracheostomy
becomes displaced
within the first 7–10 days, before a
track forms, then the tissues tend to
spring back and prevent its safe
replacement – so do not attempt to
replace it: the patient should be
reintubated.

Formal tracheostomy

A cuffed tube, usually with a removable
inner tube, is inserted by means of a
surgical operation (typically in theatre),
such that a track is formed immediately.
If the tracheostomy becomes displaced
it is often possible to open the track
and replace it.

Key point

All patients with a
formal tracheostomy
should have a
tracheostomy set, including
tracheostomy forceps, at the bedside.

Minitracheostomy

This is an uncuffed tube used primarily
to facilitate suctioning in patients with
poor cough that may be placed in
intensive care settings or occasionally on
the ward.

Complications of tracheostomies

Immediate complications include haemorrhage, direct injury to the trachea or paratracheal structures, air embolism, apnoea and cardiac arrest. Early complications are subcutaneous emphysema, pneumothorax or pneumomediastinum, tube displacement, tube blockage, infection, tracheal necrosis, and difficulty swallowing. Late complications include haemorrhage, granuloma formation, tracheocutaneous or tracheoesophageal fistula, tracheal stenosis and scarring.

Principles of tracheostomy management

> Cleaning – the biggest concern with tracheostomies is obstruction, hence it is essential that tracheostomies are kept clean; removable inner tubes should be inspected and cleaned regularly.

> Infection – the tracheostomy site should be inspected regularly and kept dry. Any moisture under the dressings will encourage skin breakdown, and infection at the site may compromise the airway.

> Humidification – inadequate humidification of inspired gas results in heat loss, moisture loss and hypoxia (functional residual capacity and static compliance fall due to atelectasis); overhumidification can result in impairment of mucociliary clearance and surfactant activity.

> Suctioning – this will stimulate the cough reflex and prevent accumulation of secretions that can cause tracheostomy blockage. Suctioning systems may be open or closed, with the latter commonly used in the ICU setting to reduce the risk of infection.

> Check cuff pressure – the inflation pressure of the cuff should be kept to a minimum to prevent trauma to the trachea, with the recommended limit being 15–25 cmH$_2$O.

Changing a tracheostomy

Percutaneous temporary tracheostomies are generally changed at around 10 days when a track has formed. Formal tracheostomies may be changed for a different size or type depending on clinical circumstances. To change a tracheostomy:

> Full resuscitation facilities should be available in case of difficulties; patients should be starved in case emergency reintubation is required; and intravenous access should be available.

> The procedure should be explained to the patient – it is mildly unpleasant and often results in coughing.

> Organise monitoring – oxygen saturation and ECG.

> Remove any oropharyngeal secretions by suction.

> Deflate the cuff of the existing tracheostomy tube and remove it.

> Insert the new tracheostomy with inner tube into the track and inflate the cuff.

> Secure the new tracheostomy tube in place.

3.8 Ventilatory support

Respiratory failure may be due to inadequate oxygenation (type 1 respiratory failure) or inadequate ventilation (type 2 respiratory failure). Type 1 can be partially or completely treated with controlled oxygen therapy or continuous positive airway pressure (CPAP), and type 2 with non-invasive positive pressure ventilation (NIPPV) or invasive positive pressure ventilation. ABGs should be obtained in all patients who are thought to have respiratory failure to determine the degree of hypoxaemia and hypercapnia and guide further management.

3.8.1 Controlled oxygen therapy

> Mild hypoxaemia (PaO$_2$ >8.0 KPa) – nasal prongs at 2–4 L/min or a Venturi mask at 24%.

> Moderate to severe hypoxaemia (PaO$_2$ 6.7–8.0 KPa) without CO$_2$ retention – simple mask with 4–15 L/min depending on ABGs.

> Moderate hypoxaemia with CO$_2$ retention – use controlled oxygen therapy using a Venturi mask. Start at 24% O$_2$ and reassess ABGs at 20 minutes. If the patient remains hypoxaemic and if the PaCO$_2$ has risen less than 1.3 KPa, increase the FiO$_2$ to 28%. Recheck ABGs. If hypoxia persists with no deterioration in CO$_2$ consider further incremental increases in FiO$_2$ with close monitoring (ABGs). If hypercapnia progresses, NIPPV or invasive positive pressure ventilation should be considered. Remember that for patients with COPD their baseline PaO$_2$ may be 7.0–8.0 KPa – are any previous blood gases available that would indicate their baseline oxygenation?

> Severe hypoxaemia (PaO$_2$ <6.7 KPa) – give high-flow oxygen via a reservoir mask and get immediate help.

> ! Hazard

Hypoxia kills quicker than hypercapnia

> All severely ill patients should receive high-flow oxygen.

> Patients with COPD who rely on their hypoxic drive for ventilation should receive high-flow oxygen initially if they are very ill. This may buy time to institute other therapies – if they improve, slowly reduce the FiO$_2$; if they do not improve, consider ventilatory support.

3.8.2 Continuous positive airway pressure

Continuous positive airway pressure (CPAP) is used in patients with acute type 1 respiratory failure when hypoxia persists despite high-flow oxygen supplementation. CPAP is helpful in improving oxygenation in patients with distal airways collapse throughout recruitment and stenting of alveoli. When using CPAP, consider the following:

> Indications – acute pulmonary oedema, pneumonia and obstructive sleep apnoea.

> Contraindications – haemodynamic instability; life-threatening hypoxia; exhaustion, impaired mental state, depressed conscious level (GCS score <8) or confusion; recent facial or upper airway surgery or facial pathology, eg burns; recent upper gastrointestinal surgery; inability to protect the airway; and copious secretions or vomitus. A chest drain needs to be inserted prior to commencing CPAP in patients with a pneumothorax.

> Practical considerations – CPAP is administered via a tight-fitting nasal or facial mask. The usual range of pressure used is 5–10 cmH$_2$O. Alterations in settings are guided by the oxygen saturations, blood gas analysis and the clinical situation. A wide-bore nasogastric tube can be inserted to enable decompression of the stomach if necessary.

> Complications – intolerance of face mask; air leaks; gastric distension; vomiting and aspiration; eye irritation and conjunctivitis; and facial skin necrosis.

3.8.3 Non-invasive ventilation

Non-invasive ventilation (NIV) refers to the use of ventilatory support via a mask or similar device. NIV is used in patients with type 2 (hypercapnic) respiratory failure. The machine is set to deliver two alternating pressures: expiratory positive airway pressure (EPAP) and inspiratory positive airway pressure (IPAP). The following points should be considered:

> Indications – NIV should be considered in patients with acute exacerbation of COPD who have respiratory acidosis (pH <7.35) despite maximal treatment; acute or acute on chronic hypercapnic respiratory failure is also an indication. Patients who are more acidotic (pH <7.26) may benefit from NIV but there is a greater risk that treatment will fail and that invasive ventilation may be required.

> Contraindications – haemodynamic instability; life-threatening hypoxia; exhaustion, impaired mental state, depressed conscious level (GCS score <8) or confusion; recent facial or upper airway surgery or facial pathology, eg burns; recent upper gastrointestinal surgery; inability to protect the airway; and copious secretions or vomitus. A chest drain needs to be inserted prior to commencing NIV in patients with a pneumothorax.

> Practical considerations – NIV is administered via a tight-fitting nasal or facial mask. EPAP should be set at 4–5 cmH$_2$O initially while IPAP should be set at 10 cmH$_2$O and rapidly increased in increments of 2–5 cm to a target of 20 cmH$_2$O. This gradual titration of pressure improves compliance. It is important that patients are closely monitored both for signs of improvement and deterioration: an ABG should be measured 1 hour after commencing treatment or after setting changes. If there appears to be clinical decline or if there is no objective improvement on NIV then invasive ventilation should be considered if appropriate.

> Complications – intolerance of face mask, air leaks and ventilator–patient asynchrony; gastric distension, vomiting and aspiration; eye irritation and conjunctivitis; and facial skin necrosis.

Key point

When initiating NIV it is important to consider the escalation plan in the event that the patient worsens despite NIV. Specifically, would invasive ventilation be appropriate?

3.8.4 Invasive ventilation

Invasive ventilation is applied via an endotracheal tube or tracheostomy. Ventilation (and therefore the PCO$_2$) is adjusted either by altering the inspiratory pressure or by changing the tidal volume directly (depending on the ventilator setting – see below). Oxygenation is improved by increasing inspired oxygen concentration or increasing the positive end expiratory pressure (which acts in a similar manner to recruit collapsed alveoli and reduce the work of breathing). When using invasive ventilation, consider the following:

Indications

The following are potential indications for invasive ventilation:

> airway protection, eg facial trauma or burns or an unconscious patient

> reversible respiratory failure (type I or type II)

> prophylactic ventilation, eg after major surgery where some degree of respiratory failure might be expected

> to avoid or control hypercapnia, eg in acute head injury or hepatic coma

> in 'flail' chest to act as an internal splint

> to facilitate the removal of secretions, eg in Guillain–Barré syndrome and myasthenia gravis.

Control of the airway

In order to secure a definitive airway, an endotracheal (ET) tube is passed through the vocal cords into the trachea. The most common method of intubation is orotracheal intubation in which a tube is passed via the mouth under visualisation using a laryngoscope. This is an extremely uncomfortable procedure which usually requires a general anaesthetic. The tube should be secured in place and it is important that the position is confirmed. This can be done immediately using a carbon dioxide detector (capnography) and auscultation to confirm bilateral air movement. If the ET tube is inserted on the ICU then the position should be confirmed on chest X-ray (the distal tip should sit around 2 cm above the bifurcation of the carina).

Occasionally nasotracheal intubation may be preferred to an orotracheal tube as it is better tolerated by the conscious patient and fixation is more secure. Its disadvantages are damage to the nasal mucosa, alar cartilages and nasal septum; bronchial suction is more difficult; and it causes an increased resistance to gas flow and an increased incidence of sinus infection.

Tracheostomy has the advantage over intubation of being better tolerated by patients, such that sedation can be reduced and weaning is often facilitated. Indications include prolonged ventilation; expected prolonged absence of protective laryngeal reflexes; retention of secretions; head and neck injuries/surgery; and upper airway obstruction. Complications include displacement of the tube, bleeding and infection; tracheal stenosis; and failure of the tracheostomy track to heal.

Modes of ventilation

Mechanical ventilation can operate under different modes. The nomenclature of these is complicated but the basic concept relies on control of the following variables:

> Volume control – this delivers a fixed tidal volume regardless of changes in lung mechanics. If the lungs become stiffer, the inflation pressure will increase to deliver the same tidal volume. This risks damage to the lungs if very high pressures are required in order to deliver the preset volume. In adults, in order to minimise ventilator-associated trauma, tidal volume is usually set at 6–7 mL/kg.

> Pressure control – delivers a preset airway pressure. If lung compliance falls or airway resistance increases then the tidal volume delivered will fall. This is the most commonly used mode in the intensive care setting. In some modes the patient is able to breathe spontaneously and this triggers the machine to deliver a breath once a certain inspiratory flow is reached.

> Respiratory rate – along with the tidal volume this will control the minute ventilation. Modes that allow patients to 'trigger' breaths should also have a built-in back-up rate which allows the minimum respiratory rate to be set.

> Inspiratory:expiratory ratio. This is commonly set at 1:2 but a more prolonged expiratory phase may be required in patients with obstructive airways disease (eg asthma) in order to minimise gas trapping.

General management of the ventilated patient

It is essential that the patient's breathing is synchronised to that of the ventilator. Failure to do so results in increased oxygen requirement, increased carbon dioxide production, reduced cardiac output and is distressing to the patient. Sedation is therefore required.

Inhaled gases should be warmed, humidified and filtered. Secretions should be cleared by regular physiotherapy and endotracheal suction. Pulse oximetry and measurement of end tidal carbon dioxide provides continuous assessment of oxygenation and ventilation, and ABGs should be checked regularly.

Complications of invasive ventilation

> Ventilator-associated pneumonia – ventilated patients have a 10–20 times increased risk of acquiring pneumonia compared with non-ventilated patients.

> Lung damage – overdistension of the alveoli and other mechanical effects may exacerbate lung injury. High inflation pressures can cause pneumothorax or subcutaneous emphysema.

> Adverse haemodynamic effects – a raised intrathoracic pressure reduces venous return and increases pulmonary vascular resistance; furthermore, cardiac output and arterial BP are reduced, and heart rate and systemic vascular resistance rise.

4 Self-assessment

4.1 Self-assessment questions

MRCP(UK) Part 1 examination questions

Question 1

Clinical scenario

A 57-year-old Asian woman presented to the emergency department with severe central chest pain. She had a past medical history of hypertension, diabetes, asthma and irritable bowel syndrome. Her medications included amlodipine, metformin, gliclazide, aspirin, montelukast and prednisolone, also salbutamol and beclometasone inhalers. Clinical examination revealed pulse 78 beats per minute, blood pressure (BP) 178/88 mmHg and a soft ejection systolic murmur. A chest X-ray showed a widened mediastinum and subsequently a computerised tomography (CT) scan revealed a type-B aortic dissection. The cardiothoracic surgical team reviewed the images and advised optimal medical management.

Question

What treatment is the most important to start?

Answer

A aspirin

B atorvastatin

C esmolol

D nitroprusside

E 0.9% saline

Question 2

Clinical scenario

A 78-year-old man was found collapsed at home with a Glasgow Coma Scale (GCS) score of 13 (E3V4M6) and a pyrexia. On examination in the emergency department he appeared drowsy and unwell, but he said that he had a headache. His observations were as follows: temperature 39.1°C, pulse 110 beats per minute, BP 85/58 mmHg, respiratory rate 22 breaths per minute, oxygen saturations 97% on air (normal range 94–98). On examination he had obvious neck stiffness and photophobia. Treatment was started with dexamethasone and ceftriaxone 2 g bd.

The next day the microbiologist called to inform the ward that they had cultured Gram-positive cocci in pairs and chains in his blood cultures and cerebrospinal fluid (CSF).

Question

Which pathogen has been cultured?

Answer

A *Haemophilus influenzae*

B *Listeria monocytogenes*

C *Neisseria meningitidis*

D *Staphylococcus aureus*

E *Streptococcus pneumoniae*

Question 3

Clinical scenario

A 79-year-old man was admitted with central chest pain. He had a past medical history of hypertension and diabetes. On the morning following admission he was witnessed by nursing staff to suddenly lose consciousness. The cardiac arrest team were called. When they arrived a defibrillator was already attached and chest compressions were in progress. The electrocardiogram (ECG) was as shown (see Fig 53). The patient had no signs of life and no palpable pulse.

Question

What is the most appropriate immediate treatment?

Answer

A defibrillation followed by assessment of ECG rhythm and pulse check

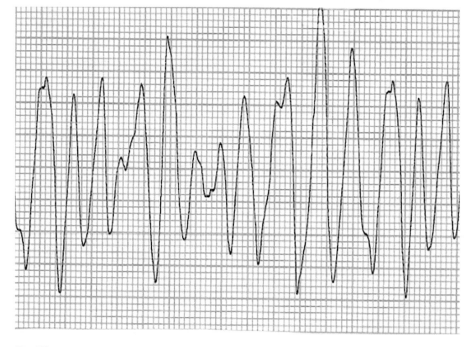

Fig 53

B defibrillation followed by immediate recommencing of cardiopulmonary resuscitation (CPR)

C establish secure airway by endotracheal intubation

D give adrenaline intravenously

E give amiodarone intravenously

Question 4

Clinical scenario

An 89-year-old woman was brought to the emergency department by ambulance having been found collapsed by her morning carers. She lived alone but had a history of dementia and her carers routinely attended four times daily. Other past medical history included paroxysmal atrial fibrillation (AF), for which she took bisoprolol and warfarin. She also took ramipril for hypertension. On arrival her observations included temperature 33.7°C, pulse 38 beats per minute, BP 105/60 mmHg, respiratory rate 14 breaths per minute and oxygen saturations 95% on air (normal range 94–98). She was conscious and appeared comfortable, but she was unable to give any history as to what happened. On examination she was peripherally cool with a slow, regular pulse. The ECG was as shown (see Fig 54).

Question

What is the most appropriate immediate management?

Answer

A atropine

B isoprenaline

C stop bisoprolol

D transcutaneous pacing

E transvenous pacing

Question 5

Clinical scenario

A 72-year-old man was brought in by ambulance to the emergency department. His wife had woken in the night to find him shaking violently. He had a past medical history of hypertension and type 2 diabetes, but he had never had seizures previously.

On the arrival of the ambulance crew, his finger-prick blood glucose was 7.5 mmol/L (normal range 3.0–6.0). They administered 10 mg rectal diazepam. On arrival in the emergency department he was still fitting. A further dose of lorazepam (4 mg IV) was given, and this was then repeated 10 minutes later. You are now called to assess him, by which time he has been fitting for 30 minutes.

Question

What treatment should be given?

Answer

A diazepam

B levetiracetam

C lorazepam

D phenytoin

E propofol

Question 6

Clinical scenario

A 58-year-old woman presented to the emergency department with a few days history of feeling generally unwell and nauseous, but with no infective symptoms. She had a past medical history of asthma, diabetes and hypertension, and was taking aspirin, amiloride, amlodipine, gliclazide, lisinopril and Symbicort as her regular medications. On examination her chest was clear and heart sounds were normal.

Her routine observations were temperature 37.1°C, pulse 98 beats per minute, BP 104/68 mmHg, respiratory rate 19 breaths per minute, oxygen saturations 97% on air (normal range 94–98). A chest X-ray was clear. An ECG was as shown (Fig 55).

Question

What biochemical abnormality is most likely to be present?

Answer

A calcium 3.30 mmol/L

B C-reactive protein (CRP) 250 mg/L

C phosphate 1.90 mmol/L

D potassium 7.5 mmol/L

E sodium 152 mmol/L

Question 7

Clinical scenario

A 72-year-old woman presented to the ambulatory care unit and was subsequently diagnosed with a pulmonary embolism. She was prescribed rivaroxaban for anticoagulation.

Question

What is the mechanism of action of rivaroxaban?

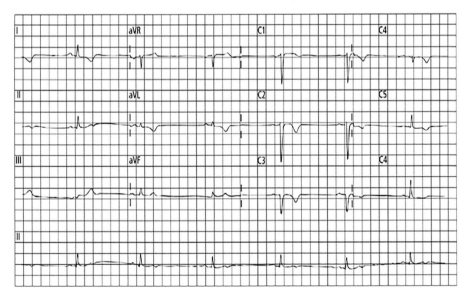

Fig 54

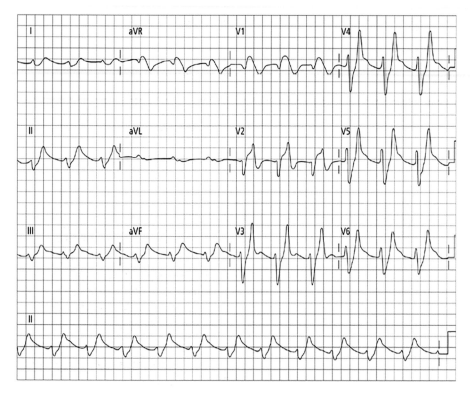

Fig 55

Answer

A direct IIa inhibitor

B direct thrombin inhibitor

C direct Xa inhibitor

D indirect IIa inhibitor

E indirect Xa inhibitor

Question 8

Clinical scenario

A 58-year-woman presented to her general practitioner (GP) for a routine check-up. Blood tests revealed serum magnesium 0.28 mmol/L (normal range 0.75–1.05).

Question

Which drug is most likely to be the cause?

Answer

A amitriptyline

B diltiazem

C lithium

D omeprazole

E ranitidine

Question 9

Clinical scenario

A 34-year-old man presented to the emergency department having taken a significant intentional overdose of amitriptyline.

Question

Which feature is typical for amitriptyline overdose?

Answer

A bradycardia

B hypersalivation

C narrow complex tachycardia

D pupillary constriction

E urinary retention

Question 10

Clinical scenario

A 40-year-old woman attended the emergency department with increased shortness of breath and wheeze. She was a known asthmatic and had been using her salbutamol inhaler a couple of

times every hour for the last 6 hours, but feeling no better. She had had three admissions in the last year with asthma exacerbations.

She was treated with nebulized salbutamol (5 mg) and ipratropium bromide (500 µg), run via oxygen, and given prednisolone 40 mg orally. She was reassessed 30 minutes later.

Question

Which sign suggests a life-threatening asthma attack?

Answer

A cannot complete sentences in one breath

B $PaCO_2$ 5.0 kPa (normal range 4.7–6.0)

C peak expiratory flow rate (PEFR) 210 L/min (predicted 420)

D pulse 120 beats per minute

E respiratory rate 25 breaths per minute

Question 11

Clinical scenario

A 74-year-old man, a heavy smoker with a 50-pack-year history but no significant past medical history, presented to the emergency department with 'noisy breathing'. The triage nurse was concerned that he had stridor and requested urgent medical review. On direct questioning he admitted that he had been unwell for the last few months, with a cough and weight loss. He had no infective symptoms, and apart from a raised respiratory rate his observations were stable.

Question

What is the most likely diagnosis?

Answer

A anaphylaxis

B aspiration of a foreign body

C epiglottitis

D laryngeal tumour

E retrosternal thyroid

Question 12

Clinical scenario

An 85-year-old man was brought to the emergency department by ambulance. His wife had noticed he had been increasingly confused and drowsy over the last few days, and called for an ambulance when she could not wake him up in the morning. She told you that apart from a few falls over the last month, he was reasonably fit for his age and taking aspirin and simvastatin as his only regular medications.

On examination he had a GCS score of 13 (E3, V4, M6). There was no focal neurology. General physical examination was unremarkable. As further investigations were being organised, the results of a venous blood gas analysis became available, with the most notable finding being plasma sodium 110 mmol/L (normal range 137–144).

Question

What is the most likely cause of hyponatraemia?

Answer

A cardiac failure

B medication

C meningitis

D prostate cancer

E subdural haematoma

Question 13

Clinical scenario

A 70-year-old woman was admitted to the stroke ward after she presented with right-sided weakness and was found to have an ischaemic left middle cerebral artery infarct on CT scan. She was diabetic, hypertensive and an ex-smoker. Four days later she was much improved and fit for discharge.

Question

Which anticoagulation/antiplatelet regimen is most appropriate?

Answer

A aspirin

B aspirin and dipyridamole MR

C clopidogrel

D dipyridamole MR

E warfarin

Question 14

Clinical scenario

A 40-year-old woman was admitted with severe cellulitis and prescribed intravenous flucloxacillin. During the infusion she complained of problems breathing and facial swelling. From the end of the bed it was clear that she had a marked degree of tongue and lip swelling, and that she had stridor. The rapid response team were called.

Question

What is the first treatment that should be given?

Answer

A adrenaline IM

B adrenaline IV

C chlorpheniramine

D hydrocortisone

E salbutamol

Question 15

Clinical scenario

A 50-year-old woman presented to the emergency department with abdominal pain. She had seen the surgical on-call team who felt that this was not a surgical problem and asked the medics to review. The patient reported that the pain had been ongoing for several weeks, and thought that it had started soon after a holiday in Malta. She described the pain as being sharp, felt in the top of her abdomen, and that it seemed to occur just before meals and overnight. Apart from taking ibuprofen for the pain she was on no medication, and she had no significant past medical history. On direct questioning she revealed her alcohol intake to be about 30 units a week, although none for the last few weeks.

On examination she had a body mass index (BMI) of 40 and was tender in her epigastrium, although there was no guarding or rebound. Bowel sounds were normal.

Question

What is the most likely diagnosis?

Answer

A biliary colic

B duodenal ulcer

C intestinal angina

D pancreatitis

E peptic ulcer disease

Question 16

Clinical scenario

A 42-year-old man presented with paroxysms of atrial fibrillation (AF), which were infrequent. He had no evidence of structural heart disease. After discussion it was decided that he would best be managed using the 'pill-in-the-pocket' strategy.

Question

What would be the most appropriate 'pill' to prescribe

Answer

A amiodarone

B bisoprolol

C digoxin

D flecainide

E propranolol

Question 17

Clinical scenario

A 65-year-old woman who was known to abuse alcohol was brought to the emergency department after she was found confused and shaking in her flat by a visiting carer. Concern was raised that she might have Wernicke's encephalopathy.

Question

What features would support the diagnosis of Wernicke's encephalopathy?

Answer

A apraxia, confusion, ophthalmoplegia

B apraxia, confusion, headache

C ataxia, confusion, headache

D ataxia, confusion, ophthalmoplegia

E confusion, headache, ophthalmoplegia

Question 18

Clinical scenario

A 78-year-old woman was brought to the emergency department by ambulance after collapsing in the street. On examination it was clear that she had sustained a stroke. She was dysphasic, with a right-sided hemiparesis.

Question

What type of stroke has she suffered?

Answer

A brain stem syndrome

B lacunar syndrome

C partial anterior circulation syndrome

D posterior circulation syndrome

E total anterior circulation syndrome

Question 19

Clinical scenario

A 48-year-old man was found collapsed in the street and brought to the emergency department. On examination he was moaning, but not speaking intelligible words. His eyes were closed, but opened to painful stimulation, and he localised to that painful stimulation.

Question

What was his GCS?

Answer

A 8

B 9

C 10

D 11

E 12

Question 20

Clinical scenario

A 58-year-old man was admitted with confusion and lethargy. General examination was unremarkable, and there were no focal neurological signs. Blood tests revealed serum corrected calcium 3.8 mmol/L (normal range 2.20–2.60).

Question

Which medication could contribute to his hypercalcaemia?

Answer

A furosemide

B lisinopril

C lithium

D omeprazole

E ranitidine

MRCP(UK) Part 2 examination questions

Question 21

Clinical scenario

A 24-year-old woman with a 3-year history of ulcerative colitis presented to the emergency department with worsening abdominal pain, diarrhoea and a pyrexia. She was opening her bowels five times per day with occasional blood and mucus mixed in.

Her observations included temperature 38.2°C, pulse 95 beats per minute, respiratory rate 16 breaths per minute, BP 110/70 mmHg, oxygen saturation 98% on air (normal range 94–98). An abdominal X-ray showed some oedema of the large bowel wall on the left side, but no dilatation. Blood test results were as follows: full blood count – normal, urea and electrolytes (U&E) – normal, liver function tests (LFTs) – normal, albumin 32 g/L (normal range 37–49), CRP 16 mg/L (normal threshold <10).

Question

Which of the patient's findings is a marker of acute severe colitis?

Answer

A abdominal X-ray findings

B albumin 32 g/L

C bowel opening five times per day

D CRP 16 mg/L

E temperature 38.2°C

Question 22

Clinical scenario

An 80-year-old man with cardiac failure, on insulin for type 2 diabetes, was admitted to hospital following a fall.

While on the ward he developed a severe hypoglycaemic attack, with a capillary blood glucose reading of 1.1 mmol/L (normal range 3.0–6.0) He was unconscious (GCS 5/15). He had no intravenous access, and it looked as though it would be very difficult to insert an intravenous cannula because of considerable peripheral oedema.

Question

What is the most appropriate next step?

Answer

A administer fruit juice orally

B administer intramuscular glucagon

C attempt to place a blue cannula in his foot for administration of intravenous dextrose

D insert a jugular central venous line for administration of intravenous dextrose

E insert a nasogastric (NG) tube for administration of fruit juice

Question 23

Clinical scenario

A 27-year-old man who had returned to the UK from a safari holiday in Zambia 3 days previously was brought to the emergency department by his wife when he developed a fever, malaise and became drowsy over the course of several hours. He had been taking mefloquine as malaria prophylaxis while travelling. On examination he looked unwell with mild hepatosplenomegaly. Venous bloods revealed a modest thrombocytopenia and raised inflammatory markers. A thick and thin film confirmed malaria with a parasite burden of 4%.

Question

What would be the most appropriate treatment?

Answer

A artemether and lumefantrine

B artesunate

C chloroquine

D doxycycline

E sulfadoxine/pyrimethamine

Question 24

Clinical scenario

A 27-year-old football supporter attended the emergency department with a minor laceration to his arm sustained in a fight. He had no medical or psychiatric comorbidities. He was assessed by an emergency physician who noted that the patient appeared to be drunk. He examined him thoroughly, documented normal observations, and identified no injury other than the laceration, which he sutured. A finger-prick blood glucose reading was 5.5 mmol/L (normal range 3.0–6.0).

The patient was waiting to go home when he became aggressive because he felt that he had waited too long for treatment. He threatened a nurse and punched a porter. You are the only other member of staff around as the rest of the medical and nursing team are dealing with a trauma call.

Question

What is the correct way to proceed?

Answer

A attempt to detain the patient under the Mental Capacity Act for assessment

B attempt to detain the patient under the Mental Capacity Act for treatment

C call hospital security and the police

D sedate the patient with intramuscular haloperidol

E sedate the patient with intramuscular lorazepam

Question 25

Clinical scenario

A 29-year-old man presented to the emergency department with a non-productive cough. He had started to feel unwell 2 days previously, with fevers and myalgia associated with a few episodes of diarrhoea. He was normally fit and well, with no significant past medical history. He had recently returned from a holiday in Turkey with his girlfriend.

His chest X-ray on admission showed right lower lobe consolidation. Blood test results included white cell count (WCC) 20.1×10^9/L (normal range 4.0–11.0) (neutrophils 15.7×10^9/L; normal range 1.5–7.0), CRP 278 mg/L (normal threshold <10) and sodium 129 mmol/L (normal range 137–144).

Question

What is the likely cause of pneumonia?

Answer

A *Haemophilus influenzae*

B *Legionella pneumophila*

C *Mycoplasma pneumoniae*

D *Staphylococcus aureus*

E *Streptococcus pneumoniae*

Question 26

Clinical scenario

A 64-year-old man presented to the emergency department with a haematemesis. His wife reported that he had vomited several bowls full of altered blood. He had also had an episode of diarrhoea, which she described as having been 'very dark'.

He had a past medical history of chronic kidney disease and type 2 diabetes, and he took aspirin, ramipril and metformin as regular medications. He denied any alcohol intake, but according to his wife used to drink heavily.

On examination there were no stigmata to suggest chronic liver disease. His observations were temperature 37.8°C, pulse 110 beats per minute, BP 105/65 mmHg, respiratory rate 16 breaths per minute, oxygen saturations 98% on air (normal range 94–98). Blood tests revealed haemoglobin 80 g/L (normal range 130–180), platelets 160×10^9/L (normal range 150–400), prothrombin time 14 s (normal range 11.5–15.5), sodium 138 mmol/L (normal range 137–144), potassium 4.9 mmol/L (normal range 3.5–4.9), urea 26.8 mmol/L (normal

range 2.5–7.0), creatinine 290 μmol/L (normal range 60–110), bilirubin 20 μmol/L (normal range 1–22), alkaline phosphatase (ALP) 150 IU/L (normal range 45–105), alanine aminotransferase (ALT) 50 IU/L (normal range 5–35).

Question

What feature is the most concerning in terms of prognosis?

Answer

A age

B blood pressure

C haemoglobin

D history of alcohol excess

E renal failure

Question 27

Clinical scenario

An 84-year-old man was referred to the admission avoidance clinic by his GP due to a finding of hypercalcaemia. He had been taken to his GP by his daughter who was concerned that he was becoming very drowsy. On direct enquiry he reported some weight loss over the last 6 months. His past medical history included hypertension for which he took amlodipine, but he was on no other medications. On examination he appeared pale and slightly thin. Repeat blood test results included haemoglobin 85 g/L (normal range 130–180), sodium 138 mmol/L (normal range 137–144), potassium 4.5 mmol/L (normal range 3.5–4.9), urea 19 mmol/L (normal range 2.5–7.0), creatinine 210 μmol/L (normal range 60–110), corrected calcium 3.20 mmol/L (normal range 2.20–2.60).

Question

Which investigation is most likely to be helpful in making a diagnosis?

Answer

A angiotensin-converting enzyme

B chest X-ray

C parathyroid hormone

D prostate-specific antigen

E serum protein electrophoresis

Question 28

Clinical scenario
A 72-year-old woman was referred to the medical admissions unit by her GP because she was not coping at home, with severe fatigue and loss of appetite. Her past medical history included breast cancer with previous mastectomy, osteoarthritis, asthma and hypertension. Her medications included paracetamol, lisinopril and amlodipine. She was accompanied by her daughter, who reported that her appetite had been poor for several weeks and that in the last 2 days she had hardly taken any food or drink. She had not opened her bowels for several days.

On examination she appeared drowsy and dehydrated, with dry mucus membranes and reduced skin turgor. Basic observations include pulse 90 beats per minute and BP 108/70 mmHg. Her jugular venous pressure (JVP) was not visible. Her abdomen was distended but soft, and there were sluggish bowel sounds. There was axillary lymphadenopathy on the same side as the mastectomy scar. Blood test results included corrected calcium level 3.5 mmol/L (normal range 2.20–2.60), urea 25.4 mmol/L (normal range 2.5–7.0) and creatinine 190 μmol/L (normal range 60–110).

Question
What should be your initial treatment?

Answer
A 0.9% saline

B 5% dextrose

C calcitonin

D pamidronate

E zoledronic acid

Question 29

Clinical scenario
A 54-year-old man presented to the emergency department with a 1-week history of progressive double vision and unsteadiness on mobilising. He had no relevant past medical history, and was on no regular medications.

On examination he had reduced sensation bilaterally and absent reflexes. His observations were normal.

Question
Which antibodies are most likely to be present?

Answer
A anti-dsDNA

B anti-gp210

C anti-GQ1b

D anti-SCL

E anti sp100

Question 30

Clinical scenario
A 62-year-old man presented to the emergency department with a severe headache that had suddenly started while he was washing a car 6 hours previously. He was otherwise well, with no relevant past medical history. On examination he was nauseous and had mild neck stiffness. There was no clinical or biochemical evidence of infection. Observations were normal. An ECG showed normal sinus rhythm and a chest X-ray was normal.

Question
Which is the most appropriate management plan?

Answer
A monitor in high dependency unit (HDU) and perform CT head at 12 hours post onset time

B perform CT head and – if normal – discharge with analgesia

C perform CT head and – if normal – perform lumbar puncture at 12 hours post onset time

D perform lumbar puncture and – if normal – discharge with analgesia

E perform lumbar puncture and – if normal – perform CT angiogram

Question 31

Clinical scenario
An 80-year-old woman presented to the emergency department less than 24 hours after a permanent pacemaker had been inserted for complete heart block. She complained of left-sided chest pain and shortness of breath. On examination, she was uncomfortable and in pain over the left side of her chest, with respiratory rate 22 breaths per minute. An ECG revealed that pacemaker spikes were present.

Question
Which would be the most appropriate investigation to do next?

Answer
A chest X-ray

B CT chest

C D-dimer

D echo

E troponin

Question 32

Clinical scenario
A 50-year-old woman with palpitations was referred to the on-take medical team by her GP. She felt that her heart beat had been faster than normal since the previous evening. She also mentioned that she had been feeling very anxious for the last few weeks and had lost some weight. Her past medical history included coeliac disease for which she observed a gluten-free diet.

Her basic observations were temp 39.5°C, pulse 145 beats per minute (regular), BP 150/85 mmHg, respiratory rate 20 breaths per minute, oxygen saturations 98% on air (normal range 94–98). On examination she was flushed and sweating with a slight tremor. Blood tests sent by her GP 1 week previously showed thyroid-stimulating hormone (TSH) 0.01 mU/L (normal range 0.4–5.0)

Question
What immediate treatment should be given?

Answer
A atenolol

B carbimazole

C digoxin

D Lugol's iodine

E propylthiouracil

Question 33

Clinical scenario

An 88-year-old woman was admitted with abdominal discomfort and a low-grade fever. Her past medical history included alcohol excess, depression, diabetes, osteoarthritis, osteoporosis and urinary incontinence. Her regular medications were calcium tablets, chlordiazepoxide, citalopram, codeine, gliclazide, paracetamol and oxybutynin. No firm diagnosis was made to explain her abdominal symptoms and fever, but she was treated with oral antibiotics.

Six days after admission you were asked to review her because she complained to the nurses that she was feeling tired and nauseous. Apart from elevated inflammatory markers and an elevated serum creatinine, her blood test results were otherwise normal on admission. Repeat blood tests revealed haemoglobin 125 g/L (normal range 115–165), white cell count (WCC) 13 × 10^9/L (normal range 4.0–11.0), potassium 4.8 mmol/L (normal range 3.5–4.9), creatinine 130 μmol/L (normal range 60–110), CRP 58 mg/L (normal threshold <10), bilirubin 10 μmol/L (normal range 1–22), ALT 890 U/L (normal range 5–35) and ALP 138 U/L (normal range 45–105).

Question

What is the most likely cause of the above results?

Answer

A alcohol

B chlordiazepoxide

C citalopram

D codeine

E paracetamol

Question 34

Clinical scenario

A 42-year-old man presented to the emergency department in a confused and drowsy state. He had a long history of excess alcohol intake, with known liver cirrhosis, and he had a 4-month history of progressive abdominal swelling. His regular medications were thiamine, vitamin B-co-strong, codeine and rifaximin.

On examination he was drowsy (GCS 12) and slow to perform commands, but with no focal neurology. His pupils were normal sized and reactive. His speech was slow, but there was no evidence of dysphasia. His chest was clear and his abdomen distended with shifting dullness.

Basic observations included temperature 38.5°C, pulse 100 beats per minute, BP 95/56 mmHg, respiratory rate 20 breaths per minute, oxygen saturations 96% on air (normal range 94–98). Investigation results included finger-prick blood glucose 5.4 mmol/L (normal range 3.0–6.0), urine dipstick (2+ leukocytes), ECG (sinus tachycardia) and chest X-ray (normal).

Question

What is the next most appropriate step in management?

Answer

A prescribe chlordiazepoxide and Pabrinex

B prescribe naloxone and stop codeine

C request CT head

D request ultrasound abdomen and insert ascitic drain

E septic screen and start antibiotics

Question 35

Clinical scenario

A 65-year-old man presented to the emergency department with a 6-hour history of severe central chest pain and sweating. He had a past medical history of diabetes, and he had suffered an ischaemic stroke 1 month previously.

His ECG was compatible with an acute ST-segment elevation myocardial infarction (STEMI), and after initial resuscitation, including 300 mg aspirin, the local percutaneous coronary intervention (PCI) service was phoned with a view to urgent transfer. Unfortunately, they reported that they had another patient in the catheter laboratory and would not be able to treat this patient for 3 hours.

Question

What is most appropriate next management step for this patient?

Answer

A Clopidogrel

B nitrate infusion

C Fondaparinux

D thrombolysis

E transfer for PCI

Question 36

Clinical scenario

A 20-year-old student with insulin-dependent diabetes was brought to the emergency department by her partner. She had been unwell for several days with a fever, abdominal pain and vomiting. She had not been measuring her blood sugars or taking her insulin for the previous 24 hours because she had felt too unwell to do so.

On examination she was febrile, tachycardic and hypotensive. Initial blood results included glucose 30 mmol/L (normal range 3.0–6.0), ketones 3.5 mmol/L (normal threshold <0.6) and potassium 5.7 mmol/L (normal range 3.5–4.9). A diagnosis of diabetic ketoacidosis was made and she was resuscitated with an appropriate fluid regimen and a variable rate insulin infusion.

Question

Under what circumstances would it be appropriate to stop the insulin infusion?

Answer

A her ketones have returned to normal

B her potassium has returned to normal

C her temperature has returned to normal

D normal blood glucose

E she is eating and drinking again

Question 37

Clinical scenario

A 50-year-old man with a past medical history of diabetes and hypertension presented to the emergency department with his wife. His wife reported that he appeared confused, with muddled speech. She said that he had been mildly unwell, with some coryzal symptoms over the last week, and had complained of a headache the previous evening. Today, when they got up in the morning, she noticed that he 'wasn't making any sense' and that he did not seem to be moving his right arm as much as normal.

Routine observations included temperature 38.5°C and BP 180/90 mmHg. On examination he had some word-finding difficulties and appeared to be confused. The power in his right arm was 3/5 and in his right leg 4/5. He was mildly tender to pressure over his sinuses. His heart sounds were normal.

Question

What is the most likely diagnosis?

Answer

A cerebral abscess

B cerebral metastasis

C encephalitis

D stroke

E subarachnoid haemorrhage

Question 38

Clinical scenario

A 22-year-old man was brought into the emergency department by the police. They had been called by his neighbours, who had found him in the garden, semi-naked and shouting. The police were concerned about his medical fitness and so had brought him to the hospital as a place of safety.

When you tried to approach he was verbally aggressive and the police reported he had been lashing out at them. You established that he has no capacity to make decisions at this time, and tried to calm him down in a

non-confrontational manner. However, despite this he continued to refuse any medical help, and you judged that he was a danger to himself, the emergency department staff, and to other patients.

Question

How would you proceed?

Answer

A ask the police to deal with him

B call security to continually restrain him

C haloperidol

D lorazepam

E lorazepam and haloperidol

Question 39

Clinical scenario

An unknown man is brought to the emergency department having been found collapsed in the street. He appeared to be in his 50s but had no identifying information on him.

His basic observations were temperature 35.8°C, pulse 95 beats per minute, BP 150/70 mmHg, respiratory rate 12 breaths per minute, oxygen saturations 95% on air (normal range 94–98). On examination his GCS was 7 (E1, V1, M5). Both pupils were reactive, but the left appeared larger than the right and was slower to react.

Question

What investigation is your immediate priority?

Answer

A arterial blood gas

B blood cultures

C blood glucose

D CT head

E electrocardiogram

Question 40

Clinical scenario

An 84-year-old man presented to the acute medicine clinic with a 2-week history of progressive shortness of breath. He was a heavy ex-smoker and had a history of chronic obstructive pulmonary disease, ischaemic heart disease and benign prostatic hypertrophy.

On examination he was cachectic, jaundiced and mildly tachypnoeic, but with a clear chest. There was no calf swelling. Observations included pulse 78 beats per minute, blood pressure 145/62 mmHg, respiratory rate 22 breaths per minute, oxygen saturations 88% on air (normal range 94–98). Blood tests revealed creatinine 92 μmol/L (normal range 60–110), bilirubin 30 μmol/L (normal range 1–22), haemoglobin 104 g/L (normal range 130–180), platelets 180×10^9/L (normal range 150–400), international normalised ratio (INR) 1.1 (normal threshold <1.4). A CT pulmonary angiogram (CTPA) showed a subsegmental embolus in the right upper lobe and a 3 cm speculated lesion in the left lower lobe.

Question

What is the next most appropriate step in his management?

Answer

A anticoagulate with low-molecular-weight heparin

B anticoagulate with rivaroxaban

C anticoagulate with warfarin

D refer for inferior vena cava filter

E withhold anticoagulation until biopsy performed

4.2 Self-assessment answers

Answer to Question 1

D: nitroprusside

Optimal blood pressure control is of paramount importance to prevent extension of the dissection flap. In most cases intravenous beta-blockade would be used, but this is not the only option and the fact that the woman is asthmatic and on multiple medications for this suggests that a nitroprusside infusion would be the best option in her case.

Answer to Question 2

E: *Streptococcus pneumoniae*

This is a classic presentation of pneumococcal meningitis in an older man, with typical microbiological findings in his cultures that make the diagnosis beyond all possible doubt. The Gram-stain microscopy of the organisms listed here are as follows:

Haemophilus influenzae – Gram-negative rod

Listeria monocytogenes – Gram-positive rod

Neisseria meningitidis – Gram negative coccus

Staphylococcus aureus – Gram-positive coccus growing in clumps

Streptococcus pneumoniae – Gram-positive coccus growing in pairs and chains.

Answer to Question 3

B: defibrillation followed by immediate recommencing of cardiopulmonary resuscitation (CPR)

The electrocardiogram (ECG) shows ventricular fibrillation (VF), which is a shockable rhythm. The priority is to administer a shock as soon as possible. Following defibrillation, CPR should be resumed immediately and the rhythm and pulse checked after the next 2 minutes unless the patient shows signs of life.

If VF / pulseless ventricular tachycardia (VT) persists following three shocks then 1 mg adrenaline and 300 mg amiodarone should be given. Endotracheal intubation may be appropriate if skilled staff are present, but should not delay defibrillation.

Answer to Question 4

C: stop bisoprolol

Her blood pressure is adequate, hence atropine, isoprenaline and pacing are not required. It is not clear whether the bradycardia caused her to collapse and alternative causes of syncope should be considered. The bisoprolol and

hypothermia may be contributing to her bradycardia. It is therefore reasonable to observe and see what her heart rate is once normothermic and without the beta-blocker. If she remains bradycardic then pacing may need to be considered, but there is no indication for this at present.

Answer to Question 5

D: phenytoin

This man has been fitting for at least 30 minutes continuously and is therefore in established status epilepticus, which has failed to respond to benzodiazepines. He should receive a loading dose of phenytoin. He will require general anaesthesia, intubation and ventilation if seizures still do not terminate.

Answer to Question 6

D: potassium 7.5 mmol/L

The patient has presented with nausea, has relatively low blood pressure for somebody who is known to be hypertensive, and is borderline tachycardic, all suggestive of dehydration. In addition, she is on an angiotensin-converting enzyme (ACE) inhibitor (lisinopril) and potassium-sparing diuretic (amiloride), which have further contributed to her developing hyperkalaemia, which is apparent from her ECG.

Answer to Question 7

C: direct Xa inhibitor

Rivaroxaban (and apixaban) are direct Xa inhibitors. Fondaparinux is an indirect inhibitor of Factor Xa. Dabigatran is a direct thrombin/IIa inhibitor.

Answer to Question 8

D: omeprazole

Long-term use of proton pump inhibitors (PPIs) has been associated with reduced magnesium and

calcium absorption, leading to hypomagnesaemia and hypocalcaemia. Loop, thiazide diuretics, cisplatin and alcoholism are also associated with hypomagnesaemia. Lithium, especially in toxic levels, is associated with hypomagnesaemia.

Answer to Question 9

E: urinary retention

If taken in sufficient quantities, amitriptyline, a tricyclic antidepressant, causes anticholinergic effects (dry mucous membranes, constipation, urinary retention, pupillary dilation) as well as cardiac arrhythmias, the most concerning of which are the broad complex tachycardias, VT and VF.

Answer to Question 10

B: PaCO$_2$ 5.0 kPa (normal range 4.7–6.0)

The other four answer options are compatible with an acute severe asthma attack, but not a life-threatening one as defined by the British Thoracic Society / Scottish Intercollegiate Guidelines Network (BTS/SIGN) guidelines. A normal PaCO2 in the context of an acute asthma attack suggests that the initial phase of low PaCO2 (associated with hyperventilation in order to maintain adequate oxygenation) has passed, and that the patient is beginning to tire. Urgent referral to the intensive care unit (ICU) is required.

Answer to Question 11

D: laryngeal tumour

The chronicity of symptoms points away from a diagnosis of aspiration of foreign body or anaphylaxis. There have been no preceding infective symptoms and the patient is 74 years old, which makes epiglottitis very unlikely. The history could be compatible with retrosternal thyroid or tumour, but in the context of heavy smoking and weight loss a malignancy has to be first on the differential.

Answer to Question 12

E: subdural haematoma

The most likely diagnosis here is that the patient has sustained a traumatic subdural haematoma (SDH) following one of his falls and this had led to him developing syndrome of inappropriate antidiuretic hormone secretion (SIADH), and his gradual onset of increased confusion and drowsiness. Careful management is required to gradually increase his sodium over the next few days, and an urgent CT head is needed to confirm the diagnosis.

Answer to Question 13

C: clopidogrel

NICE guidelines recommend clopidogrel as the preferred long-term antiplatelet therapy post stroke. If this is not tolerated or contraindicated then low-dose aspirin and dipyridamole are the alternative. Patients with atrial fibrillation (AF) should receive high-dose aspirin for 2 weeks and then formal anticoagulation.

Answer to Question 14

A: adrenaline IM

This woman has life-threatening anaphylaxis with airway compromise. While she needs all of the medications listed, the priority is to give intramuscular (IM) adrenaline.

Answer to Question 15

E: peptic ulcer disease

The description of the pain – epigastric and relieved by food – makes peptic ulcer disease the most likely diagnosis. She also has risk factors for this with high alcohol consumption and non-steroidal anti-inflammatory drug (NSAID) use. However, given her body mass index (BMI), age and the position of the pain, biliary colic should be considered, and it would be important to check the serum amylase to rule out pancreatitis.

Answer to Question 16

D: flecainide

In patients with infrequent paroxysms of AF and without ischaemic or structural heart disease a 'pill-in-the-pocket' strategy can be useful if patients are aware of symptoms and when to take the drug. Flecainide is the drug used in this circumstance.

Answer to Question 17

D: ataxia, confusion, ophthalmoplegia

Wernicke's encephalopathy is the triad of ophthalmoplegia (horizontal and/or vertical nystagmus; weakness/failure of eye abduction; and weakness/failure of conjugate gaze), ataxia and confusion. If there is a history of chronic high alcohol intake or malnutrition, give thiamine intravenously (Pabrinex) before glucose to avoid precipitating this condition.

Answer to Question 18

C: partial anterior circulation syndrome

A total anterior circulation syndrome (TACS) produces new higher cerebral dysfunction (eg dysphasia); homonymous visual field defect; and ipsilateral motor and/or sensory deficit involving at least two out of the three areas, face, arm and leg. A partial anterior circulation syndrome (PACS) produces two out of the three components of the TACS, or new higher cerebral dysfunction alone, or motor/sensory deficit more restricted than those classified as lacunar syndrome (for which, see the book text).

Answer to Question 19

B: 9

For eyes open to painful stimulation he scores E2; for moans, but no intelligible words, he scores V2; for localisation to painful stimulation he scores M5.

Answer to Question 20

C: lithium

Medications that can cause hypercalcaemia include thiazide diuretics, lithium and vitamin D analogues. Furosemide can be used in conjunction with saline infusion to treat hypercalcaemia. Lisinopril commonly causes hyperkalaemia. Milk and alkali, which were used historically to treat peptic ulcer disease, could induce hypercalcaemia, but H2-blockers and PPIs do not.

Answer to Question 21

E: temperature 38.2°C

Findings of concern in acute ulcerative colitis include bowels opening 9–12 times in the first 24 hours, a pulse rate >100 beats per minute, fever >38°C, albumin <30 g/L, C-reactive protein (CRP) >45 mg/L and mucosal islands, toxic megacolon or dilated small bowel on an abdominal radiograph.

Answer to Question 22

B: administer intramuscular glucagon

This patient has had a significant hypoglycaemic attack which needs treating urgently. It would be inappropriate to attempt oral administration of a glucose load in an unconscious patient due to the risk of causing aspiration. In addition nasogastric (NG) insertion would be challenging in an unconscious patient and it could be inserted in the wrong place. Numerous failed attempts at a challenging cannula or insertion of a central venous catheter (CVC) would simply lead to unnecessary delay.

Answer to Question 23

B: artesunate

Current UK guidelines recommend intravenous artesunate as first-line treatment for falciparum malaria with a parasite burden of greater than 2%. Notably, this is an unlicensed indication in the UK and not all centres hold this drug in stock. Intravenous quinine is recommended if there is going to be any delay in getting hold of artesunate – it is better to get started with this than accept any delay while a drug is couriered in from elsewhere.

Answer to Question 24

C: call hospital security and the police

This patient has no prior medical or psychiatric problems and there is no credible reason to suspect one now. He has simply got drunk and assaulted a member of staff in a criminal fashion. The priority should be avoiding further injury to yourself, your patients or other staff, and the most effective way to achieve this is for the police to be called. Hospital security staff are often able to provide valuable assistance before the police arrive. A criminal prosecution may be pursued in this scenario.

Answer to Question 25

B: *Legionella pneumophila*

Legionella may colonise air-conditioning systems and so should be considered in patients with pneumonia who have recently been abroad. It commonly causes a viral-like prodromal illness prior to the development of a cough. Patients may also have gastrointestinal symptoms and hyponatraemia is common.

Answer to Question 26

E: renal failure

Using the Rockall score this man has several features that put him at increased risk: age >60 years, heart rate >100 beats per minute and renal failure, giving a Rockall score of 5 prior to endoscopy (mortality 40%). The single factor that contributes most to this is the presence of renal failure (which scores 3 points).

Answer to Question 27

E: serum protein electrophoresis

The combination of hypercalcaemia with anaemia and renal impairment in an 84-year-old man is suggestive of myeloma. Investigations should include serum and urine electrophoresis, serum immunoglobulins and erythrocyte sedimentation rate (ESR).

Answer to Question 28

A: 0.9% saline

Initial treatment of hypercalcaemia should be to correct intravascular volume depletion. This woman has both clinical and biochemical evidence of dehydration and is likely to require several litres of intravenous fluid resuscitation. Once rehydrated she can be commenced on a bisphosphonate. Calcitonin is a second-line drug if there is poor response to bisphosphonates.

Answer to Question 29

C: anti-GQ1b

The presentation is that of Miller Fisher syndrome, which classically presents with the triad of ophthalmoplegia, ataxia and areflexia. It is associated with anti-GQ1b ganglioside antibodies that are also associated with Guillain–Barré syndrome with ophthalmoplegia and Bickerstaff's brain stem encephalitis.

Answer to Question 30

C: perform CT head and – if normal – perform lumbar puncture at 12 hours post onset time

The presentation is highly suspicious for a subarachnoid haemorrhage. In this case, a CT head should immediately be performed as this is diagnostic in up to 98% of cases. If normal, a lumbar puncture should be performed 12 hours after onset time in order to prevent small bleeds being missed.

Answer to Question 31

A: chest X-ray

A pneumothorax is a potential complication of cardiac pacemaker insertion and one should be suspicious if a patient complains of chest pain and/or breathlessness after this procedure.

Answer to Question 32

E: propylthiouracil

The clinical diagnosis is thyrotoxic crisis, which should be treated immediately, without delaying to wait for further laboratory results. Propylthiouracil is the preferred drug as it both blocks further synthesis of thyroid hormones and inhibits peripheral T4 to T3 conversion. However, if this is not available then carbimazole should be given instead. Lugol's iodine is started later. Supportive care is also required with treatment of pyrexia and tachycardia. Glucocorticoids should also be given.

Answer to Question 33

E: paracetamol

The bloods show a grossly elevated alanine aminotransferase (ALT). We know from the history that her bloods were normal on admission, apart from her inflammatory markers and creatinine. She is presumably of low body weight, has been on regular paracetamol since admission, and received an inadvertent paracetamol overdose.

Answer to Question 34

E: septic screen and start antibiotics

The patient has a long history of alcohol abuse with liver cirrhosis. He is currently encephalopathic, most likely due to sepsis. Your immediate management is to take full cultures (including ascitic fluid if possible) and start broad-spectrum antibiotics. He will likely require a CT head, but there is no focal neurology and this is not your immediate concern. Likewise, he is not displaying signs of alcohol withdrawal.

Answer to Question 35

E: transfer for PCI

Although it is correct to also administer clopidogrel, this is not the intervention that will reperfuse the patient's cardiac muscle. The patient's ischaemic stroke within the last 3 months means thrombolysis is contraindicated, hence even though there will be a delay of more than 90 minutes in getting the percutaneous coronary intervention (PCI), this is still the management of choice.

Answer to Question 36

A: her ketones have returned to normal

A sliding scale should be continued until the patients ketones have normalised and their metabolic acidosis has resolved. This may mean continuing the sliding scale after a patient is normoglycaemic, in which case the infusing fluid should be switched from 0.9% saline to dextrose.

Answer to Question 37

A: cerebral abscess

The history of coryzal symptoms with tender sinuses in a diabetic patient make the most likely diagnosis a cerebral abscess secondary to sinusitis. The fever and insidious onset over several hours make stroke less likely. A CT scan with contrast is required to confirm clinical suspicion.

Answer to Question 38

E: lorazepam and haloperidol

This patient lacks capacity at this time and so you must act under common law in his best interests while trying to establish the cause of his distress. De-escalating techniques have failed and you believe he is a danger to himself and others, so he needs to be sedated. The safest way to do this is to try oral sedation first, and the combination of lorazepam and haloperidol is most likely to be effective. If this is not successful you may need to try intramuscular (IM) sedation, but this has an unpredictable absorption and risks needle stick injuries. Only *in extremis*, and with the proper support present, such as someone competent to manage an airway, should intravenous sedation be attempted.

Answer to Question 39

C: blood glucose

All of the investigations listed may be relevant in an unconscious patient, but the immediate priority is to check blood glucose because hypoglycaemia is easily reversible and can be fatal or lead to permanent disability if untreated. Given the asymmetry in his pupils, he will require an urgent CT head, but this needs to be done safely – consider whether he requires a medical escort and/or anaesthetic support in view of his reduced GCS.

Answer to Question 40

A: anticoagulate with low-molecular-weight heparin

The patient is an ex-smoker with chronic obstructive pulmonary disease (COPD) and the CT pulmonary angiogram (CTPA) is suspicious for a lung cancer, which may have metastasised to the liver. Guidelines state that low-molecular-weight heparin is the most suitable option for patients with an underlying cancer. There is not enough data to comment upon the use of direct oral anticoagulants (DOACs) (rivaroxaban) in patients with cancer. A biopsy will likely be required, but this is not the immediate concern.

Index